THE COMPLETE PLANT BASED DIET COOKBOOK

Inspired 200 Easy Delicious Recipes For Nourishing And Eating Well Everyday

Sabestian Gastronomer

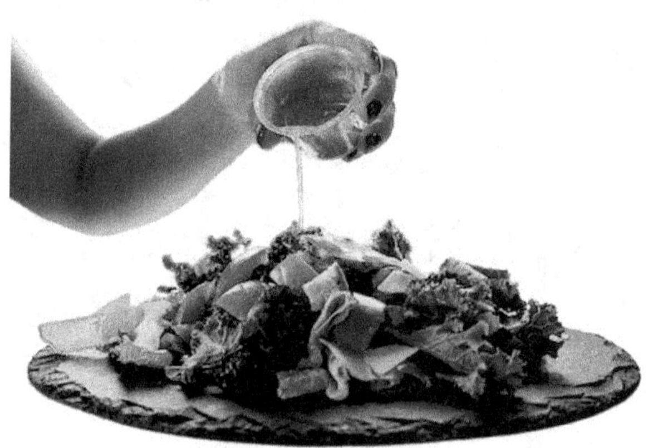

TABLE OF CONTENT

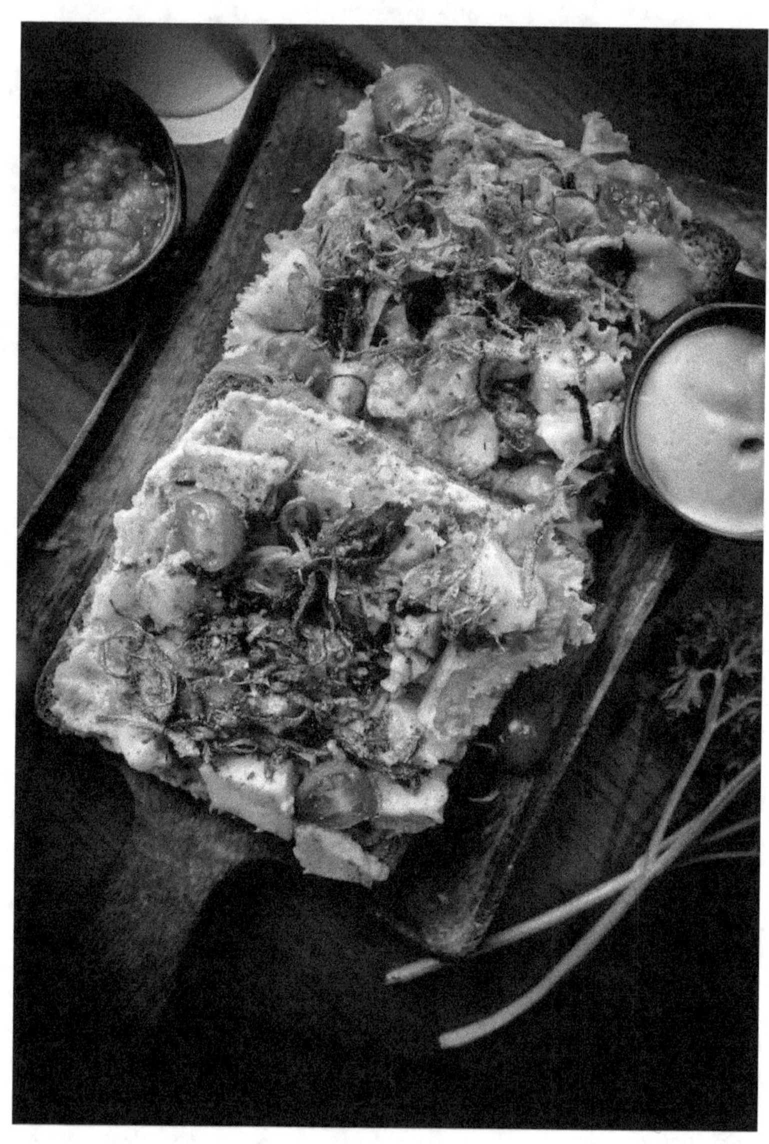

1. *"Fuel your body with the right nutrients, and it will thank you with a lifetime of vitality."*

2. *"Eating well is a form of self-respect. Treat your body with love and care."*

3. *"Your health is an investment, not an expense. Choose your food wisely."*

4. *"Healthy eating is not a diet; it's a lifestyle. Make it a habit, not a chore."*

5. *"Nourish your body, and it will nourish your soul. Good food equals a good mood."*

6. *"Every meal is an opportunity to nourish yourself. Make each choice a healthy one."*

7. *"Don't count calories; make every calorie count. Choose nutrient-dense foods for a healthier you."*

8. *"Progress, not perfection. Aim for better, not perfect, choices in your eating habits."*

9. *"The journey to a healthier you begins with the first bite. Start today, and never look back."*

10. *"You are what you eat, so why not be healthy, vibrant, and full of life? Your body deserves it!"*

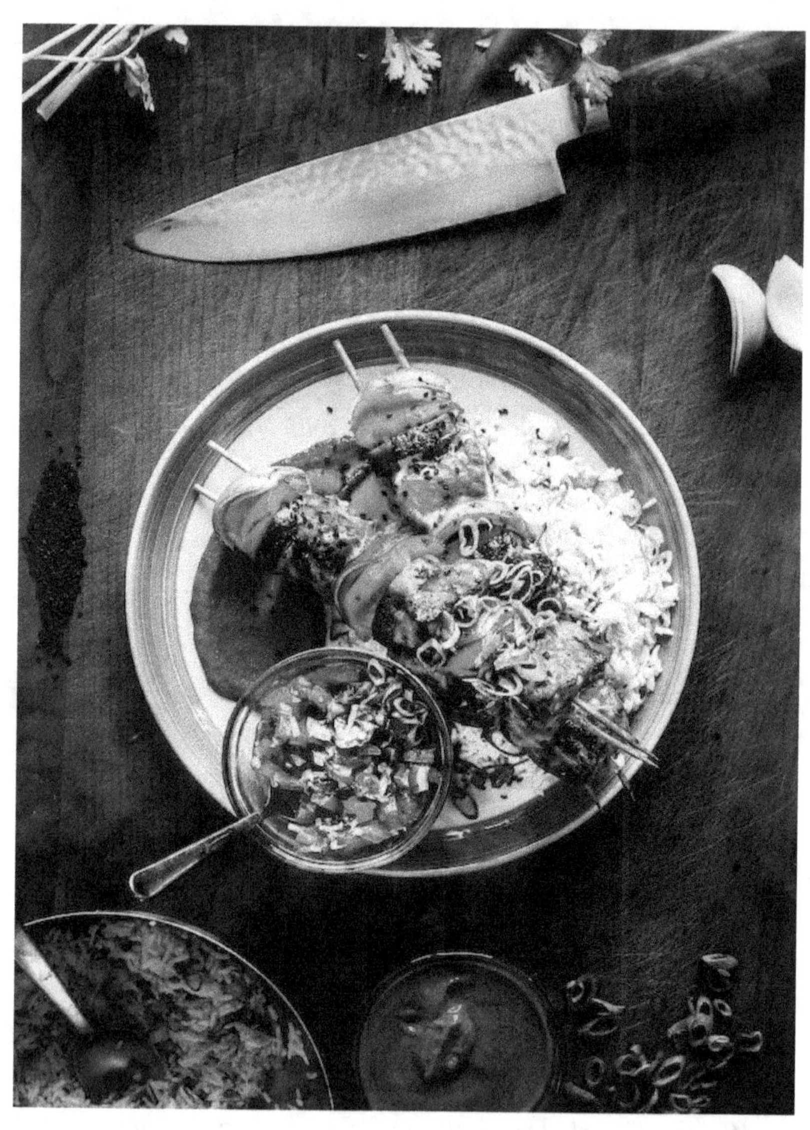

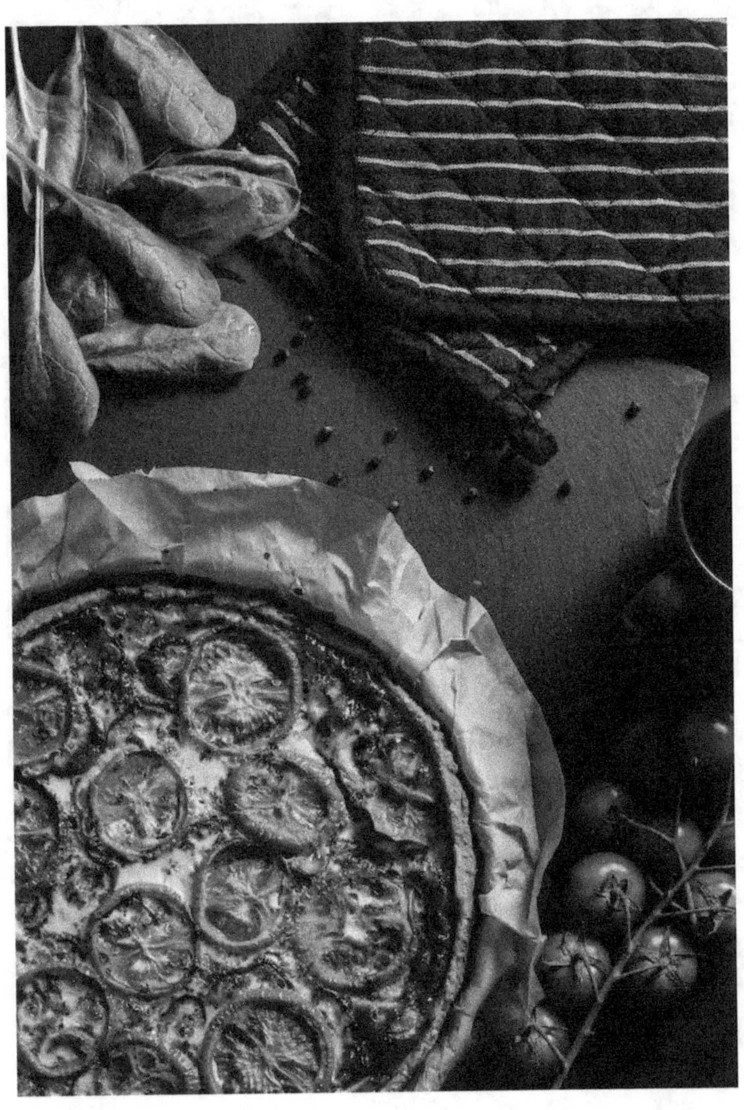

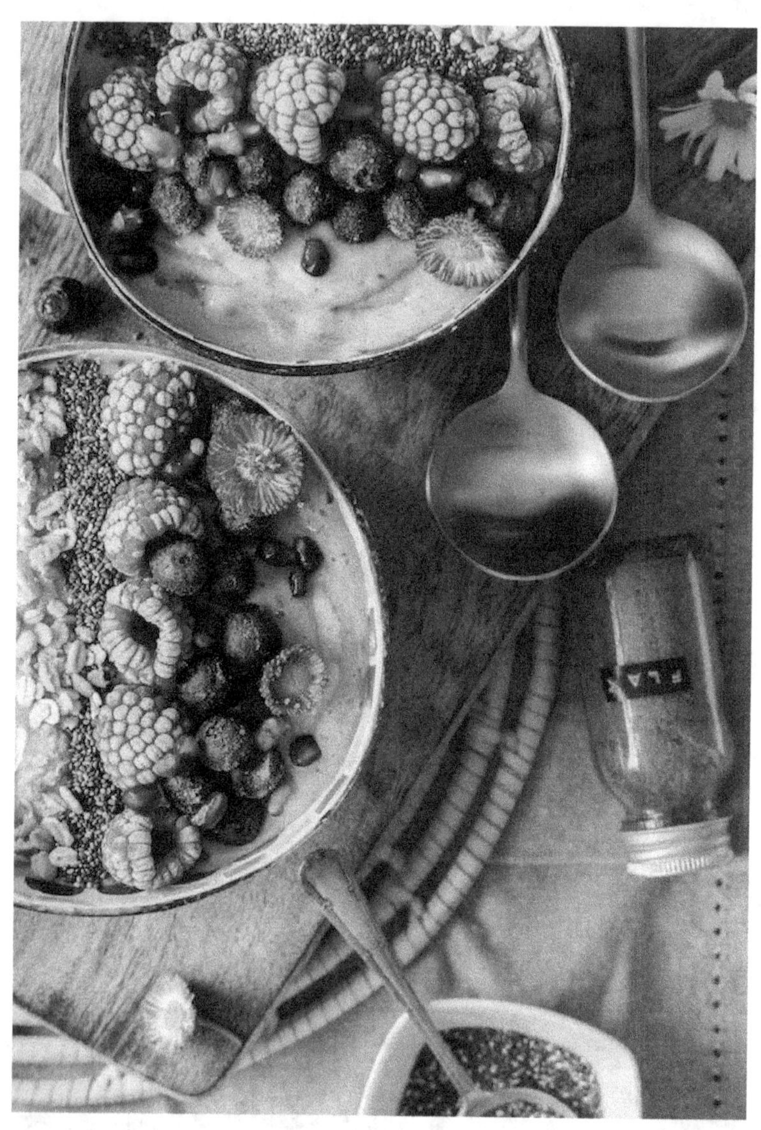

INTRODUCTION

There is a culinary revolution taking place in a world where people are becoming more sensitive to the decisions they make for their health and the environment. a movement that promotes the exciting and varied world of plant-based cooking. This cookbook is about a journey into the heart of a movement that embraces the wonderful wealth of nature and the delectable opportunities it affords, not just a collection of recipes.

Meet Emma, a passionate cook who, like many others, formerly believed that the main course should always be meat. A chance encounter with a platter of exquisitely roasted veggies, on the other hand, made her aware of the amazing tastes and sensations the plant life had to offer. She had a realization that led her to begin exploring plant-based cookery in a way she had never done before.

"The Complete Plant Based Cookbook," a cookbook by Emma, is a reflection of her culinary experience. It's an adventure full of learning, trying new things, and, most importantly, excellent cuisine. You'll discover a treasure trove of recipes in these pages, each one created to highlight the vivacious hues, varied flavors, and nourishing properties of plants. This cookbook is a celebration of the artistry that may be created using vegetables, fruits, grains, and legumes rather than merely a compilation of recipes.

You'll not only discover ideas for your next meal as you browse through these pages, but you'll also set off on a journey that will alter the way you view food. From the busy markets of Asia, where the air is filled with the aroma of herbs and spices, you will travel to the sun-drenched plains of Europe, where centuries-old culinary customs coexist with cutting-edge innovation.

"The Complete Plant Based Cookbook" invites you to go on this voyage with Emma, regardless of your level of culinary expertise. It's a voyage that will pique your curiosity about food, spark your imagination, and increase your appreciation of the wealth of nature. So put on your apron, grab a knife, and let's go on a plant-based culinary journey that will feed both your body and your soul. Welcome to a flavorful, sustainable, and delightful world.

Essential Ingredients In Plant Based Cooking

A variety of components are used in plant-based cooking to produce scrumptious and nourishing dishes. The following are some basic components frequently used in plant-based cooking:

1. Fruits and Vegetables: Fruits and vegetables are the cornerstone of plant-based cuisine and are a great source of fiber, vitamins, and minerals. To increase nutritional diversity, offer a wide variety of colorful options.

2. Legumes: A great source of protein, fiber, and several nutrients, legumes include beans (black beans, kidney beans, chickpeas), lentils, and peas. They can be used in a variety of dishes, including soups, stews, salads, and more.

3. Whole Grains: To add complex carbs, fiber, and long-lasting energy, include whole grains such brown rice, quinoa, bulgur, oats, and whole wheat pasta.

4. Nuts and Seeds: Healthy fats, protein, and texture are all provided by almonds, walnuts, chia seeds, flaxseeds, and hemp seeds. They work well as garnishes or to provide crunch and nutrition to meals.

5. Plant-Based Proteins: To increase the protein level of your foods, use tofu, tempeh, seitan, and plant-based protein powders. They can be added to smoothies and stir-fries as well as used as meat alternatives.

6. Plant-Based Milk: Almond, soy, oat, and coconut milk are among the alternatives to dairy that are utilized in dishes, cereals, and drinks.

7. Herbs and Spices: Many herbs and spices (such as basil, cilantro, oregano, turmeric, and cumin) can enhance the flavor and complexity of plant-based foods without the use of animal products.

8. Healthy Fats: Use sources of healthy fats for cooking and flavoring, such as avocados, olive oil, coconut oil, and nut butters.

9. Nutritional Yeast: A common ingredient in vegan dishes, nutritional yeast is frequently used to give food a cheesy flavor.

10. Plant-Based Sweeteners: In place of refined sugar, you can use agave nectar, maple syrup, date syrup, and coconut sugar.

11. Plant-Based Condiments: To enhance taste and depth in foods, use soy sauce, tamari, balsamic vinegar, tahini, and plant-based mayonnaise.

12. Plant-based broths and bouillon: For soups, stews, and sauces, vegetable broth or bouillon cubes are necessary.

13. Flours: Whole wheat flour, almond flour, and chickpea flour are frequently substituted for typical flours in baking and cooking.

14. Dried Fruits: Foods can benefit from the natural sweetness and texture of dried fruits like raisins, cranberries, and apricots.

15. Plant-Based Cheese: If you wish to imitate the cheesy flavor and texture in your recipes, vegan cheese alternatives are available.

16. Planet-Based Yogurt: Almond, coconut, or soy-based dairy-free yogurt can be utilized in salad dressings, desserts, and breakfast dishes.

17. Vegetable Stock: Vegetable stock is a versatile ingredient that improves the flavor of risottos, sauces, and soups.

18. Aquafaba: Also known as chickpea juice in cans, aquafaba can be whipped into a froth or substituted for eggs in baking.

19. Plant-Based Proteins: For additional protein options, consider edamame, spirulina, and nutritional powders (such as pea protein).

20. Fresh Herbs and Greens: For freshness and nutrition, include fresh herbs like parsley, cilantro, and basil as well as leafy greens like kale, spinach, and arugula.

Tips For Success

These basic components are the foundation of plant-based cooking, and there are many ways to mix them to make savory, nutrient-dense dishes that fit a vegan or vegetarian diet.

Making a smooth shift to plant-based cuisine may be rewarding and fun. Here are some pointers to help you succeed when cooking plant-based meals:

1. Educate Yourself: To make sure you're obtaining all the necessary nutrients, educate yourself on plant-based nutrition. You can make more sensible decisions if you have a basic understanding of protein, iron, calcium, and other nutrients.

2. Start Slowly: Making the switch to a plant-based diet needn't be sudden. Increase your consumption of plant-based meals to begin with, then progressively cut back on animal-based items.

3. Experiment with New Foods: Be daring and give a range of fruits, vegetables, grains, legumes, and plant-based proteins a try that you might not have previously. This can keep your food flavorful and wholesome.

4. Plan Your Meals: Make sure you have a range of ingredients on hand by planning your meals in advance. This can help you resist the urge to eat unhealthy foods when you're hurried and hungry.

5. Meal Prep: During the week, spend some time on meal preparation. To make cooking over the week easier and quicker, chop vegetables, cook grains, and make sauces or dressings in advance.

6. Learn Flavor Profiles: Knowledge of various herbs, spices, and condiments' flavor profiles can help you make delectable plant-based cuisine. Try different seasoning combinations to create your own distinctive flavors.

7. Use Fresh Ingredients: Use seasonal, fresh produce wherever possible. Compared to canned or frozen alternatives, fresh foods frequently have better flavor and nutrition.

8. Balance Your Plate: Strive to eat meals that are well-balanced and contain a variety of hues and nutrients. Vegetables, grains, legumes, and a source of protein or healthy fats should all be present on a typical plant-based diet.

9. Investigate Meat Substitutes: Tofu, tempeh, seitan, and plant-based burgers are just a few of the meat alternatives that are readily available. Try different combinations to get the flavors and textures of recipes containing meat.

10. Read Labels: When purchasing packaged foods, carefully read labels to look for substances originating from animals. Watch out for words like casein, whey, and gelatin.

11. Invest in Quality Cookware: Cooking with plants can be significantly improved by using high-quality cookware. Sharp knives, good blenders, and nonstick cookware can all be useful items.

12. Learn several cooking techniques, such as roasting, sautéing, steaming, and baking. Plant-based ingredients can exhibit distinctive flavors and textures using a variety of approaches.

13. Locate Plant-Based Alternatives: Learn about plant-based dairy substitutes like almond milk, coconut yogurt, and vegan cheese. Additionally, there are egg substitutes such as flaxseeds and chia seeds.

14. Join a Community: Look into joining a community or online organization that focuses on plant-based cuisine. You can get support on your journey, share recipes, and learn from others.

15. Stay Informed: To keep your meals interesting and motivating, stay up to date on the newest cookbooks, trends, and recipes for plant-based foods.

16. Don't Be Too Hard on Yourself: If you make a mistake or occasionally consume non-vegetarian food, try not to be too hard on yourself. The key is progress, not perfection. Every meal you choose to eat that is plant-based has a favorable effect.

17. Listen to Your Body: Keep track of how your body reacts to a plant-based diet. If you're feeling worn out or have any health issues, seek advice from a medical practitioner.

18. Enjoy the Journey: Accept plant-based cooking as a fun and creative activity. Celebrate your accomplishments and enjoy the mouthwatering flavors of your plant-based meals.

CHAPTER 1

Breakfast Delights

Toast with avocado, tomato, and basil
Ingredients:
- Whole-grain bread
- Ripe avocado
- Slices of tomato
- Fresh basil
- Salt and pepper
- Oil of olives
Prepare:
1. Crisp up the whole-grain bread as it is toasting.
2. Mash the ripe avocado in a bowl while the bread is browning.
3. When the bread is done, top it with an even layer of mashed avocado.
4. Arrange fresh basil leaves and tomato slices on top of the avocado.
5. Add a little olive oil and season to taste with salt and pepper.
6. While the avocado toast is still warm, serve it.

Vegan Pancakes
Ingredients:
- 1 cup flour,

- 1 cup vegan milk, such as almond milk
- 2 tablespoons baking powder.
- 2 tablespoons maple syrup
- 1 teaspoon vanilla extract
- A dash of salt is required.

Prepare:

1. To begin, combine the flour, baking soda, and salt in a mixing dish.

2. Combine the dry ingredients with the almond milk, maple syrup, and vanilla extract. Make sure the batter is smooth by stirring.

3. Lightly grease a nonstick griddle or pan and heat it over medium heat.

4. For each pancake, pour a ladleful of batter onto the griddle.

5. Cook the pancakes until surface bubbles appear, flip them over, and continue cooking until both sides are golden brown.

6. Top your vegan pancakes with your preferred condiments, such as nut butter, fresh fruit, or maple syrup.

Chia Pudding with Berries

Ingredients:

- 1 cup of almond milk (or any other plant-based milk)
- 3 tablespoons of chia seeds.
- 1 tablespoon of maple syrup (modify to taste)
- 1/2 teaspoon vanilla extract

- Mixed berries
- A few thinly sliced almonds, if desired

Prepare:

1. To begin, mix the chia seeds, almond milk, vanilla essence, and maple syrup in a bowl.

2. Stir thoroughly, making sure the chia seeds are dispersed equally.

3. To make the mixture thicken, place the mixture in the refrigerator for several hours or overnight.

4. When your chia pudding is ready to be served, top it with a lot of mixed berries and, if you like, some nut slices.

The Tofu Scramble

Ingredients:

- Crushed firm tofu
- Nutritional yeast
- Bell peppers
- Onions
- Spinach.
- Pepper and salt

Prepare:

1. To begin, sauté the bell peppers, onions, and garlic in a pan until they are soft.

2. Add nutritional yeast and turmeric to the pan with the crushed tofu.

3. Continue cooking until the tofu is well cooked and resembles scrambled eggs.

4. Add spinach and stir until wilted.

5. Add salt and pepper to the food to taste.

Smoothie Bowl:
Ingredients:
- Almond milk (or other plant-based milk)
- Frozen mixed berries
- Bananas.
- Chia seeds
- Spinach
- Your choice of toppings (granola, almonds, seeds, or fruit).

Prepare:
1. Blend a ripe banana, a handful of spinach, almond milk, and frozen mixed berries until smooth.
2. Put the smoothie inside a bowl.
3. Add your preferred toppings, such as granola, almonds, seeds, or fresh fruit, along with the chia seeds.

Banana and almond butter over oats:
Ingredients:
- Ripe banana
- Almond milk or any other plant-based milk.
- Rolled oats.
- Peanut butter
- Maple syrup
- Cinnamon

Prepare:
1. Prepare rolled oats with almond milk as directed on the package.
2. Cut a ripe banana into slices and stir it into the cooked oats.
3. Add a drizzle of almond butter, a dash of cinnamon, and a little maple syrup to taste for sweetness.
4. After combining everything, enjoy your creamy oatmeal.

Vegan breakfast tacos:
Ingredients:
- Black beans
- Avocado
- Salsa
- Sautéed peppers
- Sautéed onions
- Whole-grain tortilla.
- Scrambled tofu

Prepare:
1. Spread a tortilla made of whole grains.
2. Add salsa, sautéed peppers, onions, black beans, sliced avocado, and a big scoop of tofu scramble to it.
3. Fold the sides in and roll it up into a burrito to serve.

Quinoa Breakfast Bowl
Ingredients:
- 1 cup vegan milk, such as almond milk

- Cooked quinoa
- Banana slices
- Chopped nuts (such as walnuts and almonds)
(Maple syrup)
- Citron

Prepare:

1. To make quinoa creamy, combine it with almond milk.

2. Add chopped nuts, maple syrup, cinnamon, banana slices, and banana slices on top.

Vegetarian French Toast

Ingredients:

- Whole-grain bread slices
- Chickpeas flour
- 1 cup vegan milk, such as almond milk
-- Vanilla extract
-- Cinnamon
- (Maple syrup)
- Fruits in season, like berries

Prepare:

1. To make a batter, stir together chickpea flour, almond milk, cinnamon, vanilla essence, and a little bit of maple syrup in a bowl.

2. Using a griddle, fry bread slices till golden brown by dipping them in the batter.

3. Add extra maple syrup drizzles and fresh fruit to your serving.

Banana Toast with Peanut Butter
Ingredients:
- Whole-grain bread
- Peanut butter, or any other nut butter
- Sliced banana
- Cinnamon sprinkled on top
Prepare:
Toasted whole-grain bread should be crunchy when prepared.
2. Cover the toast with peanut butter
3. Add sliced banana and a dash of cinnamon on top.

Vegan Benedict with tofu:
Ingredients:
- Half an English muffin
- Sliced tomato
- Steaming asparagus
- Sautéed spinach
- Vegan hollandaise sauce
- Silken tofu (to be used in the sauce)
- Nutritional yeast
- Color-enhancing turmeric
- Citrus juice
- Pepper and salt
Prepare:
1. Toast half an English muffin.
2. Add sliced tomato and steamed asparagus or sautéed spinach to each side of the sandwich.

3. Blend silken tofu, nutritional yeast, turmeric, lemon juice, salt, and pepper until smooth to make vegan hollandaise sauce.

4. Cover the muffin halves with the sauce and serve.

Vegan breakfast tacos
Ingredients:
- Tortillas made with corn or whole grains
- Tofu scrambled with spices and turmeric.
- Salsa
- Guacamole
- Chopped cilantro
- Optionally, sliced jalapenos

Prepare:
1. Warm up the tortillas in a dry skillet.

2. If you like it spicy, add sliced jalapenos to each tortilla along with salsa, guacamole, chopped cilantro, and scrambled tofu.

3. Add a squeeze of lime juice to your vegan breakfast tacos before serving.

Vegan blueberry muffins
Ingredients:
- 1 1/2 cups all-purpose flour
- 1/2 cup whole wheat flour
- 1/2 cup sugar,
- 2 teaspoons baking powder.
- 0.5 teaspoon baking soda

- 1/2 teaspoon salt
- 1 cup vegan milk, such as almond milk
- 1/4 cup of unsalted applesauce
- 1/4 cup of heated coconut oil
- 1 tsp vanilla essence
- 1 cup blueberries, either fresh or frozen

Prepare:

One step in preparation is to line a muffin pan with paper liners and preheat the oven to 375°F (190°C).

2. Combine the flours, sugar, baking soda, baking powder, and salt in a large mixing basin.

3. Combine the almond milk, applesauce, melted coconut oil, and vanilla extract in another bowl.

4. Combine the dry components with the wet ingredients by pouring them into each other.

5. Slowly incorporate the blueberries.

6. Spoon approximately 2/3 of the batter into each muffin cup.

7. Bake the muffins for 18 to 20 minutes, or until a toothpick inserted in the center comes out clean.

8. Before serving, allow the muffins to cool.

Vegan breakfast burrito bowl

Ingredients:

- Black beans
- Cooked brown rice or quinoa
- Sautéed bell peppers and onions
- Sliced avocados

- Salsa
- Fresh cilantro
- Lime wedges are the ingredients.

Prepare:

1. Cooked brown rice or quinoa should be layered in a bowl or on a platter.
2. Add bell peppers, onions, and black beans on top.
3. Include ripe avocado slices.
4. Top with your preferred salsa.
5. To add a flavorful kick, garnish with fresh cilantro and serve with lime wedges.

Vegan overnight oats

Ingredients:

- 1 cup vegan milk, such as almond milk
- Rolled oats
- The Chia seed
- Fresh fruit (such as berries, banana slices, or maple syrup)
- Nuts and seeds, such as flax seeds and almonds

Prepare::

1. Combine rolled oats, almond milk, chia seeds, and, to taste, a drizzle of maple syrup or agave nectar in a jar or other container.
2. Give everything a good stir, making sure the oats and chia seeds are completely submerged.
3. Top with your preferred fresh fruit, nuts, or seeds.
4. Refrigerate the container overnight after sealing it.

5. Your overnight oats will be ready to eat in the morning. Stir them up quickly, then dig in!

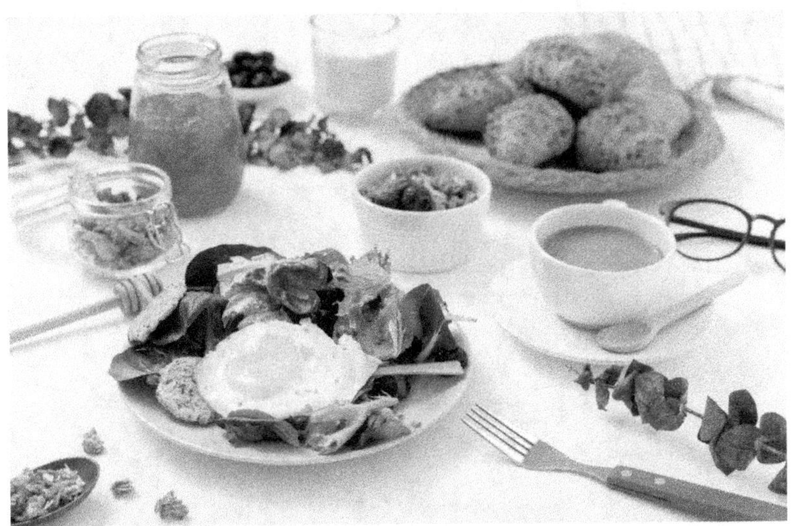

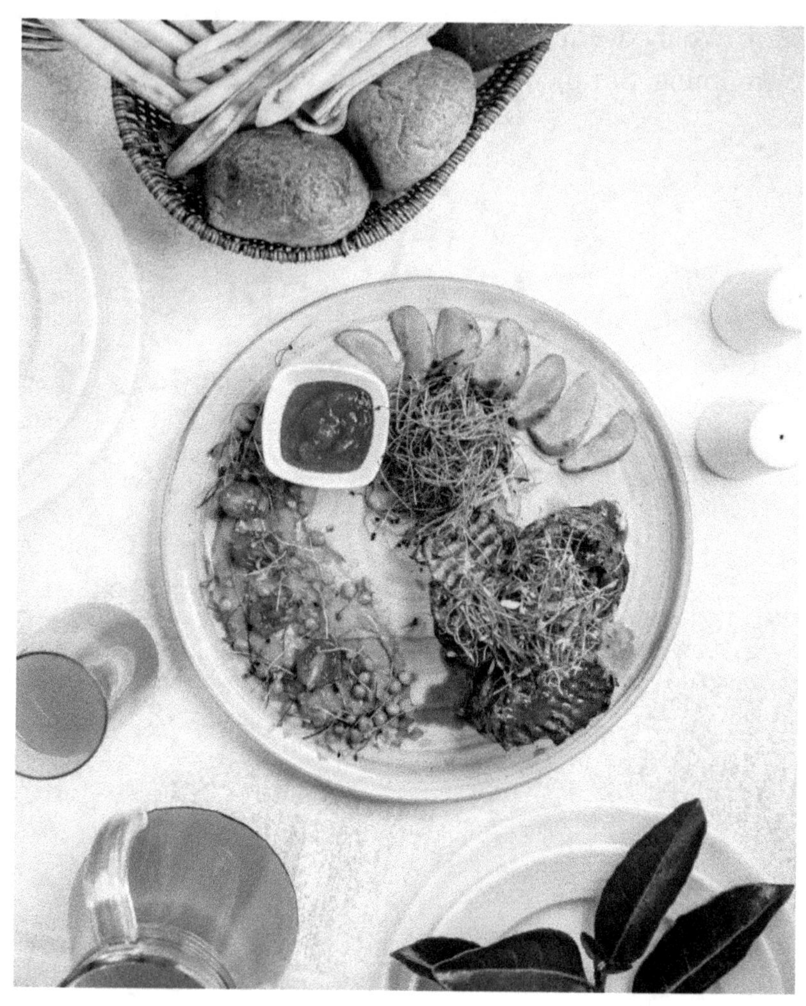

CHAPTER 2:

Appetizer And Snacks

Guacamole with Tortilla Chips:
  - **Ingredients:**
    - 2 ripe avocados
    - A single tiny red onion, chopped
    - 2 cloves garlic, minced
    - 1-2 tomatoes, diced
    - Juice of 1 lime
    - Salt and pepper to taste
  - **Prepare:** Mash avocados, mix in the rest of the ingredients, and serve with tortilla chips.

Hummus and Veggie Platter:
  - **Ingredients:**
    - 1 can chickpeas, drained
    - 2-3 tbsp tahini
    - 2 cloves garlic
    - Juice of 1 lemon
    - Salt and olive oil
    - Assorted raw veggies (carrots, cucumbers, bell peppers)
  - **Prepare:** Blend chickpeas, tahini, garlic, lemon juice, salt, and olive oil until smooth. Serve with veggies.

Stuffed Mushrooms:
  - **Ingredients:**
    - 12 large mushroom caps
    - 1/2 cup breadcrumbs
    - 1/4 cup vegan cream cheese
    - 2 cloves garlic, minced
    - Fresh parsley, chopped
  - **Prepare:** Remove mushroom stems, mix breadcrumbs, vegan cream cheese, garlic, and parsley. Stuffed mushroom caps, bake at 350°F (175°C) for 20 minutes.

Sweet Potato Fries:
  - **Ingredients:**
    - 2 sweet potatoes, cut into fries
    - 2 tbsp olive oil
    - 1 tsp paprika
    - 1/2 tsp garlic powder
    - Salt and pepper
  - **Prepare:** Toss sweet potato fries with olive oil, paprika, garlic powder, salt, and pepper. Bake at 425°F (220°C) until crispy.

Cauliflower Buffalo Wings:
  - **Ingredients:**
    - 1 cauliflower head, cut into florets
    - 1 cup flour (or chickpea flour for gluten-free)
    - 1 cup water

- 1 tsp garlic powder
- 1 tsp paprika
- Buffalo sauce
- **Prepare:** Dip cauliflower in batter, bake at 450°F (230°C) until golden, then toss in buffalo sauce.

Salsa and Homemade Pita Chips:
- **Ingredients:**
  - Whole wheat pita bread
  - Olive oil
  - Salt
  - 2 tomatoes, diced
  - 1/2 red onion, finely chopped
  - 1 jalapeño, minced
  - Fresh cilantro, chopped
  - Lime juice
- **Prepare:** Cut pita into triangles, brush with olive oil and salt, then bake at 350°F (175°C) until crispy. Serve with salsa.

Stuffed Bell Peppers:
- **Ingredients:**
  - Mini bell peppers
  - Vegan cream cheese
  - Chopped chives
- **Prepare:** Cut the tops off mini bell peppers, stuff with vegan cream cheese mixed with chives.

Cucumber Avocado Rolls:
  - **Ingredients:**
    - Cucumber slices
    - Avocado slices
    - Red bell pepper strips
    - Hummus
  - **Prepare:** Lay out cucumber slices, add avocado, red pepper, and a dollop of hummus, then roll them up.

Spinach and Artichoke Dip:
  - **Ingredients:**
    - 1 cup cooked and chopped spinach
    - 1 can artichoke hearts, drained and chopped
    - 1 cup vegan cream cheese
    - 1/2 cup vegan mayo
    - 1/4 cup nutritional yeast
  - Preparation: Mix all ingredients, bake at 350°F (175°C) until bubbly.

Vegan Spring Rolls:
  - **Ingredients:**
    - Rice paper wrappers
    - Thin rice noodles
    - Fresh mint leaves
    - Sliced avocado
    - Sliced cucumber
    - Carrot matchsticks

  - **Prepare:** Dip rice paper in warm water to soften, then fill with noodles, mint, avocado, cucumber, and carrot. Roll tightly.

Edamame with Sea Salt:
  - **Ingredients:**
    - Edamame pods
    - Sea salt
  - **Prepare:** Boil edamame pods, drain, and sprinkle with sea salt.

Roasted Red Pepper and Walnut Dip:
  - **Ingredients:**
    - 2 red peppers, roasted (from a jar)
    - 1/2 cup walnuts
    - 2 cloves garlic
    - Lemon juice
    - Salt and pepper
  - **Prepare:** Blend each item until it is smooth.

Mango Salsa:
  - **Ingredients:**
    - 2 ripe mangoes, diced
    - 1/2 red onion, finely chopped
    - 1/2 red bell pepper, diced
    - Fresh cilantro, chopped
    - Lime juice
  - **Prepare:** In a bowl mix all the ingredients.

Baked Zucchini Fritters:
  - **Ingredients:**
    - 2 zucchinis, grated and squeezed dry
    - 1/2 cup breadcrumbs
    - 1/4 cup nutritional yeast
    - 2 cloves garlic, minced
    - Fresh basil, chopped
  - **Prepare:** Mix ingredients, shape into patties, and bake until golden.

Vegan Onion Rings:
  - **Ingredients:**
    - Onion rings
    - 1 cup flour
    - 1 cup sparkling water
    - Paprika
    - Salt and pepper
  - **Prepare:** Dip onion rings in batter, then fry until golden.

Kale Chips:
  - **Ingredients:**
    - Kale leaves, torn into bite-sized pieces
    - Olive oil
    - Nutritional yeast
    - Salt

- Prepare: Toss kale with olive oil, nutritional yeast, and salt. Bake at 300°F (150°C) until crispy.

Cucumber Cups with Tzatziki:
  - Ingredients:
    - Mini cucumber cups
    - Vegan tzatziki (made with cucumber, dairy-free yogurt, garlic, and dill)
  - Prepare: Fill cucumber cups with tzatziki.

Vegan Deviled Potatoes:
  - Ingredients:
    - Baby potatoes
    - Vegan mayo
    - Dijon mustard
    - Pickle relish
    - Paprika
  - Prepare: Boil potatoes, cut in half, scoop out centers, mix with vegan mayo, mustard, and relish. Fill potato halves and sprinkle with paprika.

Sesame Ginger Snap Peas:
  - Ingredients:
    - Snap peas
    - Sesame oil
    - Soy sauce
    - Fresh ginger, minced
    - Sesame seeds

- **Prepare:** Sauté snap peas in sesame oil, add soy sauce, ginger, and sesame seeds.

Vegan Nachos:
- **Ingredients:**
    - Tortilla chips
    - Vegan cheese sauce
    - Black beans
    - Sliced jalapeno
    - Sliced olives
    - Guacamole

-ños, olives, and bake until the cheese is bubbly. Top with guacamole.

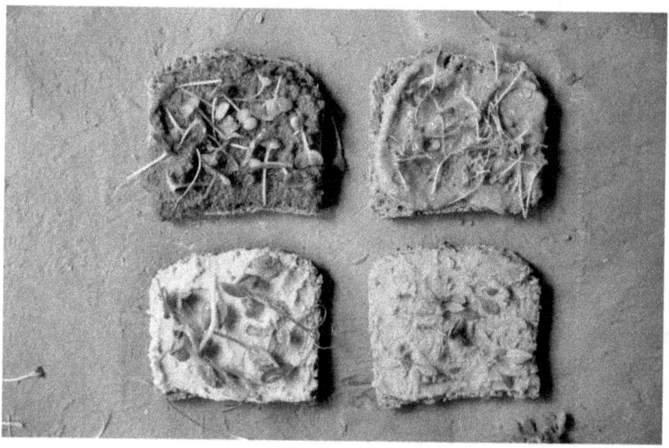

CHAPTER 3:

Salads And Desserts

A traditional garden salad dressed with balsamic vinaigrette
Salad ingredients include:
- Cherry tomatoes
- Mixed greens (lettuce, spinach, and arugula)
- Sliced cucumber
- Shredded carrots and thinly sliced red onion
- Croutons, if desired

Ingredients in dressing:
- 1 teaspoon Dijon mustard
- 1 chopped garlic clove
- 3 tablespoons balsamic vinegar
- 2 tablespoons olive oil
- To taste, salt and pepper

Preparation:
1. In a big bowl, mix the ingredients for the salad.
2. Stir the dressing ingredients in a separate bowl until thoroughly blended.
3. Pour the salad dressing over it, stir, and serve.

A vegan Caesar salad with vegan Caesar dressing
Salad ingredients include:
- Romaine lettuce

- croutons
- optional vegan parmesan cheese

Ingredients in dressing:
- Half a cup vegan mayo
- Lemon juice, 2 tablespoons
- 2 minced garlic cloves
- 1 teaspoon capers
- 1 tablespoon Dijon mustard
- One tablespoon vegan Worcestershire sauce
- To taste, salt and pepper

Preparation:
1. Combine Romaine lettuce, croutons, and any vegan Parmesan cheese you're using in a salad.
2. Blend all dressing ingredients in a blender until well-combined.
3. Add the dressing to the salad and thoroughly toss.

Quinoa salad with Mediterranean flavors

Salad ingredients include:
- Cooked quinoa
- Halved cherry tomatoes
- Diced cucumber
- Finely chopped red onion
- Pitted and sliced Kalamata olives
- Chopped fresh parsley
- Drain and washed canned chickpeas

Ingredients in dressing:
- 2 tablespoons lemon juice

- 3 tablespoons olive oil
- 1 tsp. dried oregano
- To taste, salt and pepper

Preparation:

1. In a big bowl, combine all the salad ingredients.

2. Combine the dressing ingredients in a bowl, then drizzle it over the salad. Combine by tossing.

A salad with spinach, strawberries, and poppy seed dressing

Salad ingredients include:

- Sliced fresh strawberries
- Fresh spinach leaves
- A thinly sliced red onion
- Toasted almonds
- Diced avocado

Ingredients in dressing:

- 1 tablespoon Dijon mustard
- 3 tablespoons maple syrup
- 2 teaspoons apple cider vinegar
- 3 tablespoons poppy seeds
- To taste, salt and pepper

Preparation:

1. In a bowl, combine the salad's components.

2. Stir the dressing ingredients in a separate bowl until thoroughly blended.

3. Pour the dressing over the salad and toss just enough to combine.

Peanut Noodle Salad with Thai Influence
Salad ingredients include:
- Cooked rice noodles
- thinly sliced bell peppers
- julienned carrots
- thinly sliced cucumber
- edamame beans
- freshly chopped cilantro
- Chopped peanuts
Ingredients in dressing:
- 2 teaspoons soy sauce
- 1/4 cup peanut butter
- 2 tablespoons rice vinegar
- 1 tablespoon maple syrup
- 1 minced garlic clove
- To taste, Sriracha or chili paste
- Water (to dilute)
Preparation:
1. Combine the salad's ingredients in a big bowl.
2. Combine all dressing ingredients in a another bowl and whisk until combined. To reach the correct consistency, add water as necessary.
3. Spread the salad with the peanut dressing and toss to combine.

Salad of roasted beets and walnuts with a lemon-tahini dressing

Salad ingredients include:

- Sliced roasted beets and mixed greens

- Toasted and chopped walnuts

- Thinly sliced red onion

- Optional vegan feta cheese

Ingredients in dressing:

- 2 tablespoons lemon juice

- 3 tablespoons tahini

- 1 minced garlic clove

- Water (to dilute)

- To taste, salt and pepper

Preparation:

1. Place the salad's components on a platter.

2. In a bowl, whisk the ingredients for the dressing. Add water gradually to get the appropriate consistency.

3. Dress the salad with the tahini dressing before serving.

Asian Cucumber Salad with Sesame Ginger Dressing.

Salad ingredients include:

- Thinly sliced English cucumber

- Thinly sliced red bell pepper

- Thinly sliced red onion

- Chopped fresh cilantro

- Sunflower seeds

Ingredients in dressing:

- 1 teaspoon grated ginger

- 3 tablespoons rice vinegar
- 2 tablespoons soy sauce
- 1 tablespoon sesame oil
- 1 tablespoon maple syrup
- 1 clove minced garlic

Preparation:

1. In a bowl, combine the salad's components.

2. In another bowl, combine the dressing's components.

3. After adding the dressing, gently toss the salad. Before serving, top with sesame seeds.

Chickpea Greek Salad

Salad ingredients include:

- Drained and washed canned chickpeas
- Halved cherry tomatoes
- Diced cucumber
- Finely chopped red onion
- Pitted and sliced Kalamata olives
- Chopped fresh parsley
- Vegan feta cheese (optional)

Ingredients in dressing:

- 1 teaspoon dried oregano
- 2 tablespoons red wine vinegar
- 3 tablespoons of olive oil.
- To taste, salt and pepper

Preparation:

1. In a bowl, combine all the salad ingredients.

2. Combine the dressing ingredients in a bowl, then drizzle it over the salad. Well, toss.

Black Bean and Corn Salad with Mexican Influence
Salad ingredients include:
- Drained and washed canned black beans
- Cooked and cooled corn kernels
- Halved cherry tomatoes
- Diced red bell pepper
- Diced avocado
- fresh cilantro
- freshly chopped red onion

Ingredients in dressing:
- 1 teaspoon cumin
- Salt and pepper to taste
- 3 tablespoons lime juice
- 2 tablespoons olive oil

Preparation:
1. In a big bowl, combine the salad ingredients.
2. In another bowl, combine the dressing's components.
3. Pour the dressing over the salad and toss just enough to combine.

Creamy Vegan Waldorf Salad Dressing
Salad ingredients include:
- Diced apples
- Thinly sliced celery
- Halved grapes

- Chopped walnuts
- Romaine lettuce
Ingredients in dressing:
- Half a cup vegan mayo
- Lemon juice, 2 tablespoons
- One spoonful of maple syrup.
- To taste, salt and pepper
Preparation:
1. In a bowl, combine the salad's components.
2. In another bowl, combine the dressing's components.
3. Drizzle the salad with the creamy dressing and give it a little stir.

Salads with roasted sweet potatoes and quinoa with lemon-tahini dressing.
Salad ingredients include:
- Cubes of roasted sweet potato
- Cooked quail
- Baby spinach leaves,
- Toasted and chopped pecans
- Pomegranate seeds, inoa
- Finely sliced red onion.
Ingredients in dressing:
- 2 tablespoons lemon juice
- 3 tablespoons tahini
- 2 tablespoons of water
- 1 minced clove of garlic
- To taste, salt and pepper

Preparation:

1. In a big bowl, mix the ingredients for the salad.

2. Combine the dressing ingredients in a another bowl and stir until combined.

3. Dress the salad with the lemon-tahini dressing and toss thoroughly.

Salad with Summer Berries with Balsamic Reduction.

Salad ingredients include:

- Mixture of greens
- Sliced strawberries
- The blueberry
- The blackberry
- Thinly sliced red onion
- Candied pecans

Ingredients in dressing:

- 2 teaspoons of maple syrup
- 1/2 cup of balsamic vinegar
- To taste, salt and pepper

Preparation:

1. Place the salad's components on a platter.

2. Simmer maple syrup and balsamic vinegar in a small saucepan until they become a reduction in consistency.

3. Drizzle the salad with the balsamic reduction and serve.

Roasted cauliflower salad with a lemon-Dijon dressing.

Salad ingredients include:

- Arugula

- Roasted cauliflower florets

- Halved cherry tomatoes

- Thinly sliced red onion

- Toasted and chopped almonds

- Vegan Parmesan cheese (optional)

Ingredients in dressing:

- 2 tablespoons lemon juice

- 3 tablespoons olive oil

- 1 tsp. Dijon mustard

- 1 chopped garlic clove

- To taste, salt and pepper

Preparation:

1. Combine the salad's ingredients in a big bowl.

2. In another bowl, combine the dressing's components.

3. Add the salad to the lemon-Dijon dressing and gently stir.

Asian-inspired cabbage salad

Salad ingredients include:

- Julienned carrots

- Thinly sliced green onions

- Edamame beans

- Sesame seeds

- Shredded Napa cabbage
- Red cabbage

Ingredients in dressing:
- 2 tablespoons soy sauce
- 3 teaspoons rice vinegar
- 1 tablespoon each of sesame oil and maple syrup
- 1 minced garlic clove
- 1 teaspoon of ginger, grated

Preparation:
1. In a big bowl, combine the salad ingredients.
2. In another bowl, combine the dressing's components.
3. Dress the salad with the sesame-ginger dressing and mix thoroughly.

Roasted vegetable salad with pesto dressing.

Salad ingredients include:
- Roasted veggies (such as cherry tomatoes, bell peppers, and zucchini).
- Mixture of greens
- Thinly sliced red onion
- Toasted pine nuts

Ingredients in pesto dressing include:
- 2 tablespoons pine nuts
- 1/2 cup fresh basil leaves
- 2 tablespoons nutritional yeast
- 2 tablespoons olive oil
- 1 minced clove of garlic
- To taste, salt and pepper

Preparation:
1. Place the salad's components on a platter.
2. Blend or process the ingredients for the pesto dressing until they are well-combined.
3. Toss the salad with the pesto dressing and serve.

These recipes for plant-based salads and dressings offer a range of tastes and ingredients to keep your meals flavorful and intriguing. Enjoy!

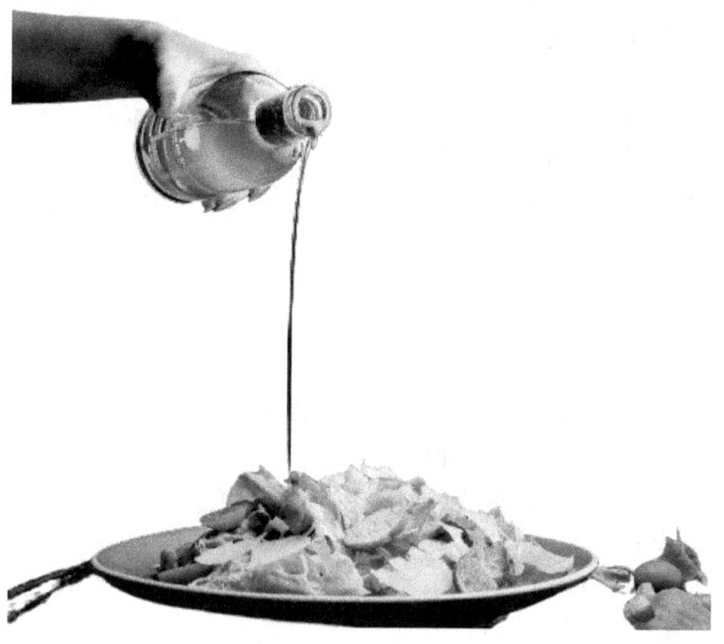

CHAPTER 4

Soups And Stews

Minestrone Soup
Ingredients:
- 1 cup diced white beans
- 1 cup diced celery
- 1 cup diced carrots
- 1 cup diced zucchini
- 1 cup diced onion
- 2 minced garlic cloves
- 4 cups vegetable broth
- 1 cup pasta.
-2 tablespoons olive oil
- Season with salt and pepper to taste
- Top with fresh basil

Instructions:
1. In a big pot, heat the olive oil. Make translucent onions and garlic by sautéing them.
2. Include tomatoes, zucchini, celery, and carrots. For five minutes, cook.
3. Add veggie broth and heat through. Simmer the pasta and beans until the pasta is done.
4. Taste-test and add salt and pepper. Before serving, garnish with fresh basil.

Lentil Soup
Ingredients:
- 1 chopped onion
- 1 cup dried green or brown lentils
- 2 sliced carrots
- 2 chopped celery stalks
- 3 minced garlic cloves
- 6 cups of vegetable broth
- 1 teaspoon each of cumin and paprika
- Add salt and pepper to taste.
- Add fresh parsley as a garnish.

Instructions:
1. Rinse the lentils, then reserve them.
2. In a sizable pot, soften the onion, carrots, celery, and garlic.
3. Include vegetable broth and lentils. Boil for a few minutes before simmering for 30 to 40.
4. Add salt, pepper, paprika, and cumin. Add fresh parsley as a garnish.

Tomato Basil Soup
Ingredients:
- 6 diced tomatoes
- 1 chopped onion
- 3 minced garlic cloves
- 1 cup of fresh basil leaves
- 4 cups of vegetable broth
-2 tablespoons olive oil

- Add salt and pepper to taste
- Optional: Add 1/2 cup coconut milk for creaminess

Instructions:

1. Get your pot of olive oil hot. Make translucent onions and garlic by sautéing them.

2. After adding, simmer the diced tomatoes for 10 minutes.

3. After adding the broth, boil the mixture for 20 minutes.

4. Blend the soup until it is smooth, then add fresh basil. If desired, stir in coconut milk.

Potato Leek Soup

Ingredients:

- four sliced leeks
- four chopped potatoes.
- 6 cups vegetable broth
- 2 minced cloves of garlic
-2 tablespoons olive oil
- Season with salt and pepper to taste
- Garnish with fresh chives

Instructions:

1. Leeks and garlic should be softened in olive oil in a big pot.

2. Include vegetable broth and diced potatoes. Till potatoes are soft, simmer.

3. Puree the soup using an immersion blender until it is smooth.

4. Add fresh chives as a garnish and season with salt and pepper.

Butternut Squash Soup
Ingredients:
- 1 diced butternut squash,
- 1 chopped onion
- 3 minced garlic cloves.
- 4 cups vegetable broth
- 2 tablespoons of olive oil
- 1 teaspoon of nutmeg
- Season with salt and pepper to taste
- Garnish with roasted pumpkin seeds

Instructions:
1. Get your pot of olive oil hot. Make translucent onions and garlic by sautéing them.
2. Include vegetable broth and butternut squash. Simmer the squash until it's tender.
3. Puree the soup with an immersion blender. Add nutmeg, salt, and pepper after that.
4. Add roasted pumpkin seeds as a garnish.

Moroccan chickpea stew
Ingredients:
- 2 cups cooked chickpeas
- 1 chopped onion
- 2 sliced carrots
- 2 diced bell peppers

- 3 minced garlic cloves
- 1 tsp coriander
- 2 tsp cumin
- 1 teaspoon paprika
-1 tomato dice from a can
- 4 cups of veggie broth
- salt and pepper to taste
- Garnish with fresh cilantro.

Instructions:

1. In a big pot, soften bell peppers, carrots, onions, and garlic.

2. Include paprika, coriander, and cumin. one more minute of cooking.

3. Add the vegetable broth, chickpeas, and diced tomatoes. For 20 minutes, simmer.

4. Add salt and pepper to taste. Add fresh cilantro as a garnish.

Mushroom Barley Soup
Ingredients:
- Two cups of sliced mushrooms
- Two diced carrots
- 1 chopped onion
- 2 chopped celery stalks
- One cup of pearl barley
- 6 cups vegetable broth
- 3 minced cloves of garlic
-2 tablespoons olive oil

- To taste-tested salt and pepper
- Garnish with fresh thyme

Instructions:

1. In a skillet over medium heat, soften the onions, garlic, carrots, celery, and mushrooms.

2. Include vegetable broth and pearl barley. 45 minutes to simmer.

3. Add salt and pepper to taste. Spritz some fresh thyme on top.

Thai Coconut Curry Soup

Ingredients:

- One can of coconut milk
- 2 tablespoons red curry paste
- 4 cups of vegetable broth
- 1 sliced cup of mushrooms
- 1 cup of sliced bell peppers
- 1 cup cubes of tofu
- 1 cup of sliced zucchini
-2 tablespoons soy sauce
- 1 teaspoon minced ginger
- 1 teaspoon minced lemongrass
-1 tablespoon lime juice
- Garnishment of fresh cilantro

Instructions:

1. Put coconut milk, vegetable broth, and red curry paste in a pot and heat. Simmer for a while.

2. Include bell peppers, zucchini, tofu, and mushrooms. The vegetables should be cooked until soft.
3. Add the lime juice, soy sauce, ginger, and lemongrass.
4. Before serving, garnish with fresh cilantro.

Black Bean Soup
Ingredients:
- 2 cans of rinsed and drained black beans
- 1 chopped onion
- 2 minced garlic cloves
- 1 diced red bell pepper
- 4 cups vegetable broth
- 2 teaspoons of cumin
- 1 teaspoon of chili powder
- Add salt and pepper to taste
- Add fresh cilantro as garnish

Instructions:
1. In a pot, soften red bell pepper, onions, and garlic.
2. Include cumin, chili powder, vegetable broth, and black beans. For 20 minutes, simmer.
3. Puree the soup using an immersion blender until it is smooth.
4. Add salt and pepper to taste. Add fresh cilantro as a garnish.

Soup with Spinach and White Beans
Ingredients:
- 1 chopped onion

- 2 diced carrots
- 2 diced celery stalks
- 2 minced garlic cloves
- 2 cans of rinsed and drained white beans
- 4 cups vegetable broth
- 2 tablespoons olive oil
- 4 cups fresh spinach
- Season with salt and pepper to taste
- Garnish with lemon wedges

Instructions:

1. Soften celery, carrots, onions, and garlic in olive oil.

2. Include vegetable broth and white beans. Steady for 15 seconds.

3. Add freshly chopped spinach and stir until wilted.

4. Add salt and pepper to taste. Serve with a lemon squeeze.

Kale and Sweet Potato Soup

Ingredients:

- 2 diced sweet potatoes
- 1 chopped onion
- 3 cups chopped kale
- 4 cups vegetable broth
- 2 minced garlic cloves.
-2 tablespoons olive oil
- 1 teaspoon paprika
- Season with salt and pepper to taste
- Garnish with toasted pumpkin seeds

Instructions:
1. In olive oil, sauté garlic and onions until they are transparent.
2. Include paprika, kale, sweet potatoes, and vegetable broth. Until sweet potatoes are cooked through, simmer.
3. Puree the soup using an immersion blender until it is smooth.
4. Add salt and pepper to taste, garnish with toasted pumpkin seeds.

Red lentil curry stew
Ingredients:
- 1 cup red lentils
- 1 chopped onion
- 2 minced garlic cloves
- 2 sliced carrots
- 2 cups tomatoes, diced
- 2 tablespoons curry powder
- 4 cups of vegetable broth
- 1 teaspoon turmeric
- Add salt and pepper to taste
- Add Fresh cilantro as a garnish

Instructions:
1. In a pot, soften the carrots, onions, and garlic.
2. Include turmeric, curry powder, red lentils, diced tomatoes, and vegetable broth. For 20 minutes, simmer.
3. Add salt and pepper to taste. Add fresh cilantro as a garnish.

Quinoa and Vegetable Stew
Ingredients:
- 1 cup rinsed quinoa
- 1 chopped onion
- 2 minced garlic cloves.
- 2 sliced carrots
- 2 chopped celery stalks
- 2 cups tomatoes, diced
- 1 teaspoon Italian seasoning
- 4 cups vegetable broth
- Add salt and pepper to taste
- Add fresh parsley as a garnish

Instructions:
1. In a pot, soften carrots, celery, onions, and garlic.
2. Include the Italian seasoning, quinoa, chopped tomatoes, and vegetable broth. For 20 minutes, simmer.
3. Add salt and pepper to taste. Add fresh parsley as a garnish.

Wild rice and mushroom soup
Ingredients:
- Two cups of sliced mushrooms
- 1 chopped onion
– One cup of wild rice
- 4 cups vegetable broth
- 2 minced cloves of garlic
-2 tablespoons olive oil
- 1 teaspoon thyme

- Add salt and pepper to taste
- Add fresh parsley as a garnish

Instructions:

1. In olive oil, soften mushrooms, onions, and garlic.

2. Include vegetable broth and wild rice. Cook the rice for 45 minutes or until tender.

3. Add the thyme, pepper, and salt. Add fresh parsley as a garnish.

Roasted vegetable stew

Ingredients:

- 1 onion, chopped
- 2 cups diced potatoes
- 2 cups diced carrots
- 2 cups diced bell peppers
- 2 cups diced eggplant.
- 3 minced garlic cloves,
- 4 cups vegetable broth
- 1 tsp rosemary
- 2 tbsp olive oil
- Season with salt and pepper to taste
- Top with fresh basil

Instructions:

1. Combine olive oil, garlic, rosemary, salt, and pepper with the diced veggies. Roast until soft in the oven at 400°F (200°C).

2. Saute onions in a pot until they are transparent.

3. Include vegetable broth and roasted veggies. Cook for ten minutes.

4. Garnish with fresh basil before serving

Thai Tom Yum Soup
Ingredients:
- 4 cups vegetable broth
- 2 thinly sliced stalks of lemongrass
- 3 slices of ginger for galangal
- 3 kaffir lime leaves
- 2 sliced tomatoes
- 1 cup sliced mushrooms
- 1 sliced onion
- 2 minced garlic cloves
-2 tablespoons soy sauce
- 1 teaspoon chile paste, taste-adjusted
- 1 teaspoon sugar
- wedges of lime as a garnish
- Garnishment of fresh cilantro

Instructions:
1. Bring vegetable broth to a boil in a pot. Add kaffir lime leaves, ginger or galangal, and lemongrass. 5 minutes of simmering.

2. Add garlic, onion, mushroom, tomato, and onion. The vegetables should be cooked until soft.

3. Add sugar, chili paste, and soy sauce.

4. Add fresh cilantro and lime wedges as garnish.

Roasted Red Pepper and Tomato Soup
Ingredients:
- 2 cans chopped tomatoes
- 4 red bell peppers, roasted and peeled
- 1 chopped onion
- 2 minced garlic cloves
- 4 cups of vegetable broth
- 2 tablespoons of olive oil
- 1 teaspoon paprika
- Season with salt and pepper to taste
- Top with fresh basil

Instructions:
1. Get your pot of olive oil hot. Make translucent onions and garlic by sautéing them.
2. Include diced tomatoes, roasted red peppers, and vegetable broth. For 20 minutes, simmer.
3. Puree the soup using an immersion blender until it is smooth.
4. Add salt, pepper, and paprika to taste. Fresh basil is a good garnish.

Mediterranean Chickpea Stew
Ingredients:
- 2 cans of rinsed and drained chickpeas
- 1 chopped onion
- 2 minced garlic cloves
- 1 cup tomatoes, diced
- 1/2 cup chopped Kalamata olives

- 1 cup chopped spinach
- 4 cups vegetable broth
- 2 tablespoons of olive oil
- 1 teaspoon of oregano
- Add salt and pepper to taste
- Add Fresh parsley as a garnish

Instructions:

1. In olive oil, sauté garlic and onions until they are transparent.

2. Include spinach, oregano, chopped tomatoes, chickpeas, and vegetable broth. Spend 15 minutes simmering.

3. Add Kalamata olives and stir. Add salt and pepper to taste.

4. Add fresh parsley as a garnish.

Mexican Black Bean Stew
Ingredients:
- 2 cans of rinsed and drained black beans
- 1 chopped onion
- 2 minced garlic cloves
- 1 sliced bell pepper
- 1 cup of kernelized corn
- 2 teaspoons of chili powder
- 4 cups of vegetable broth
- Fresh cilantro for garnish
- Salt and pepper to taste
- 1 teaspoon cumin

Instructions:

1. In a pot, soften the bell pepper, onions, and garlic.

2. Include maize, black beans, cumin, chili powder, and vegetable broth. Spend 15 minutes simmering.

3. Add salt and pepper to taste. Add fresh cilantro as a garnish.

Potato and Cabbage Soup

Ingredients:

- 1 head of shredded cabbage
- 4 diced potatoes
- 1 chopped onion
- 4 cups of vegetable broth
- 2 minced garlic cloves.
- 1 teaspoon caraway seeds
- 2 tablespoons olive oil
- To taste-tested salt and pepper
- Fresh dill for decoration

Instructions:

1. In olive oil, sauté garlic and onions until they are transparent.

2. Include the caraway seeds and cabbage shreds. Cook the cabbage until it wilts.

3. Add the vegetable broth and potato dice. Till potatoes are soft, simmer.

4. Add salt and pepper to taste. Add some fresh dill as garnish.

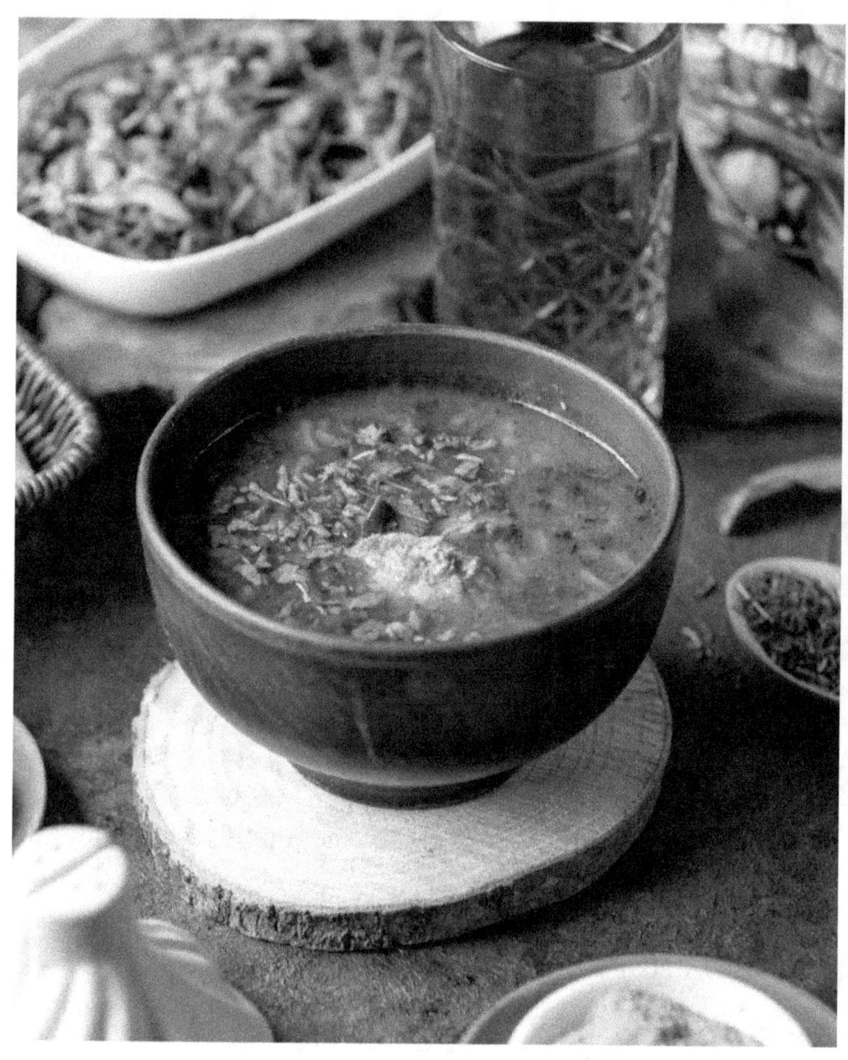

CHAPTER 5

Main Courses

Stir-fried vegetable
Ingredients:
- A variety of veggies, including carrots, snap peas, bell peppers, and broccoli.
- Cubed tofu or tempeh
-2 tablespoons soy sauce
1-tablespoon sesame oil
- 1 teaspoon minced ginger
- 2 minced garlic cloves
- Cooked noodles or rice

Preparation:
- In sesame oil, stir-fry tofu or tempeh until golden. Place aside.
- Vegetables, ginger, and garlic should be stir-fried until crisp-tender.
- Return the tofu or tempeh to the pan and mix in the soy sauce.
- Put cooked rice or noodles on top.

Vegetarian Stroganoff
Ingredients:
- 8 ounces of sliced mushrooms
- 1 cup of diced onion

- 2 minced garlic cloves
- 1 cup of coconut milk
- 1 cup of vegetable broth
- 2 tablespoons each of flour and nutritional yeast
- Cooked pasta
- Taste-tested salt and pepper

Preparation:

Mushrooms, onion, and garlic should be sautéed until the mushrooms release moisture.

- Add coconut milk, nutritional yeast, flour, and vegetable broth.

- After that add salt and pepper to simmer until sauce thickens.

- Put cooked pasta on top.

Vegetarian scrambled tofu

Ingredients:

- 1 block crumbled tofu
- 1/2 diced bell pepper
- 1/2 diced onion
- 1 teaspoon each of cumin and turmeric
- To taste-added salt and pepper
- Optional spinach or greens

Preparation:

- Soften bell pepper and onion in a skillet.

- Add salt, pepper, cumin, turmeric, and crumbled tofu.

- Tofu should be thoroughly roasted and just barely crunchy.

- Add kale or spinach and simmer until wilted.

Vegetarian enchiladas with sweet potatoes and black beans

Ingredients:
- 1 can (15 oz) washed and drained black beans
- 2 big sweet potatoes, diced
- 1 diced onion
- 2 minced garlic cloves
- One 10-ounce can of enchilada sauce
- Eight tortillas
- Vegan cheese, if desired
- Garnishment of fresh cilantro

Preparation:
Roast sweet potatoes in the oven until done.
- Garlic and onion should be sautéed until translucent.
- Combine black beans, sautéed onions, and garlic with the sweet potatoes.
- Place the mixture in a baking dish, top with enchilada sauce, and bake until cooked all the way through. Roll the mixture in tortillas.
- You can choose to add vegan cheese and bake it until it melts. cilantro is a good garnish.

Veggie Peanut Noodles in Thai Style

Ingredients:
- Rice noodles, 8 oz.
- A serving of peanut butter

-2 tablespoons soy sauce

1-tablespoon lime juice

- Add 2 teaspoons Sriracha sauce, to taste

- Broccoli florets, 1 cup

- 1 sliced red bell pepper

- 1 julienned carrot

- chopped peanuts and cilantro as garnish

Preparation:

- Prepare rice noodles as directed on the packaging.

Combine peanut butter, soy sauce, lime juice, and Sriracha in a bowl.

- Sauté the carrot, bell pepper, and broccoli until they are soft.

- Combine cooked noodles with peanut sauce and sautéed vegetables.

- Add chopped cilantro and peanuts as a garnish.

Vegan Eggplant Parmigiana

Ingredients:

- Two huge, round-cut eggplants

- One cup of breadcrumbs.

- Marinara sauce, 1 cup

- A serving of vegan mozzarella cheese

- Nutritional yeast, 1/4 cup

- Fresh leaves of basil

- Frying with olive oil

Preparation:

Slices of eggplant should be breadcrumb-coated before being fried in olive oil till golden.

- Arrange slices of eggplant, marinara sauce, vegan mozzarella, and nutritional yeast in a baking dish.

- Bake until bubbling and the cheese is melted.

- Add fresh basil leaves as a garnish.

Vegan tacos made with cauliflower

Ingredients:

- 1 head of cauliflower ,divided into florets
- 2 tablespoons taco seasoning
- Eight little corn tortillas
- Shredded lettuce, salsa, and guacamole for sprinkling

Preparation:

Cauliflower florets are roasted till soft after being tossed with taco spice.

Fill tortillas that have been heated with roasted cauliflower.

- Add salsa, guacamole, and lettuce shredded on top.

Bowl of vegan quinoa and black beans

Ingredients:

- 1 cup cooked quinoa
- 1 can (15 oz) drained and rinsed black beans
- 1 cup of kernelized corn
- 1/4 cup chopped cilantro
- 1 diced red bell pepper

- Citrus juice
- Add Slices of avocado as a garnish
  Preparation:
Cooked quinoa, black beans, corn, red bell pepper, and cilantro should all be combined.
  - Add lime juice for seasoning.
  - Add avocado slices on top.

Vegan Jackfruit Sandwich with BBQ
  Ingredients:
 - Two (20 oz) cans of shredded young green jackfruit in brine
  - 1 chopped onion
- 2 minced garlic cloves
  -1 cup barbecue sauce
  - Rolls or buns for hamburgers
  - Coleslaw as a garnish
  Preparation:
  - Sauté garlic and onion until they are tender.
  - Stir in the BBQ sauce and shredded jackfruit, and heat through.
  - Serve with coleslaw and hamburger buns.

Vegan quesadillas with mushrooms and spinach
  Ingredients:
  - 8 tiny tortillas made with whole wheat
  - 2 cups chopped mushrooms
  - 2 cups spinach

- 1 cup shredded vegan cheese
    - Cooking with olive oil
  Preparation:
Mushrooms and spinach should be sautéed until wilted.
    - Combine sautéed mushrooms, spinach, and vegan cheese on quesadillas.
    - Till cheese is melted and tortillas are crispy, cook in a pan.

Chickpea and Sweet Potato Curry, a vegan dish

Ingredients:

- 1 can (15 oz) washed and drained chickpeas
- 2 big sweet potatoes, diced
- 1 chopped onion
- 2 minced garlic cloves
- One 14-ounce can of coconut milk
- 2-tablespoon curry powder
- Add salt and pepper to taste
- Add fresh cilantro as garnishing

Preparation:

- Sauté garlic and onion until they are transparent.
- Include coconut milk, curry powder, salt, and pepper together with sweet potatoes and chickpeas.
- Simmer sweet potatoes until they are fork-tender.

Serve with rice or naan and garnish with fresh cilantro.

Vegan Stuffed Shells with Spinach and Mushrooms
Ingredients:
- 16 cooked large pasta shells
- 2 cups chopped spinach
- 2 cups chopped mushrooms
- Tofu, nutritional yeast, garlic powder, and salt make up one cup of tofu ricotta.
- Two cups of marinara sauce
- Topping of vegan mozzarella cheese

Preparation:
- Sauté spinach and mushrooms until they are soft.
- Combine sautéed vegetables with tofu ricotta.
- Stuff the mixture into cooked pasta shells.
- Place in a baking dish, top with vegan mozzarella and marinara sauce.
- Bake until bubbling and the cheese is melted.

Vegetarian Loaf of Lentils
Ingredients:
- Two cups of cooked green or brown lentils
- one diced onion
- Two minced garlic cloves
- 1 shredded carrot
- 1 cup breadcrumbs
- 1/4 cup of ketchup
-2 tablespoons soy sauce
- 1 teaspoon thyme
- To taste, salt and pepper

Preparation:

- Sauté the carrot, onion, and garlic until they are tender.

- Combine cooked lentils, ketchup, soy sauce, thyme, salt, and pepper with sautéed vegetables.

- Put the mixture in a loaf pan, then bake it until it is hard.

Vegetarian aglio e olio spaghetti

Ingredients:

- 8 ounces of whole wheat spaghetti
-4 minced garlic cloves
- To taste, add red pepper flakes to 1/4 cup of olive oil
- Freshly chopped parsley
- lemon zest
- To taste, salt and pepper

Preparation:

- Prepare pasta as directed on the package.

- Garlic and red pepper flakes are sautéed in hot olive oil until aromatic.

- Season the cooked spaghetti with salt, pepper, parsley, and lemon zest before tossing it in the garlic oil.

Vegan Shepherd's Pie with Mushrooms and Lentils

Ingredients:

- 1 cup cooked green or brown lentils
- 2 cups chopped mushrooms
- 1 diced onion

- 2 minced garlic cloves
- 1 cup of frozen carrots and peas
- 2 cups of potatoes mashed
- Salt and pepper to taste
- Vegan butter for mashed potatoes

Preparation:

- Sauté garlic and onion until they are transparent.

Mushrooms should be added and cooked until browned.

- Add cooked lentils, frozen peas, and carrots to the mixture.

- Add mashed potatoes on top, transfer mixture to a baking dish, and bake until potatoes are brown.

Vegetarian Spinach and Chickpea Curry

Ingredients:

- 2 cans (15 oz) of washed and drained chickpeas.
- 2 cups spinach
- 1 diced onion
- 2 minced garlic cloves
- 1 (14 oz) container of chopped tomatoes
- 1 (14 oz) can of coconut milk
2-tablespoon curry powder
- To taste, salt and pepper

Preparation:

- Garlic and onion should be sautéed until translucent.
- Add the curry powder, salt, pepper, coconut milk, spinach, diced tomatoes, and chickpeas.

- Simmer until chickpeas are thoroughly warm and spinach has wilted.

Vegan Bolognese with Mushrooms and Walnuts
Ingredients:
- 2 cups chopped mushrooms
- 1/2 cup chopped walnuts
- 8 oz whole wheat spaghetti
- 1 diced onion
- 2 minced garlic cloves
- 1 can (14 oz) chopped up tomatoes
  2 tablespoons tomato paste
-1 teaspoon of dried oregano
- To taste, salt and pepper

Preparation:
- Garlic and onion should be sautéed until translucent.
- Cook the walnuts and mushrooms together until the mushrooms release moisture.
- Add the tomato paste, oregano, salt, and pepper along with the smashed tomatoes.
- Put cooked spaghetti on top.

Portobello mushroom burgers that are vegan
Ingredients:
- Four substantial portobello mushroom caps
- four whole wheat hamburger buns
- Baby spinach or arugula, 1 cup
- 1 sliced tomato

- One-half of a red onion, finely sliced
- Your favorite vegan sauce
Preparation

- Balsamic vinegar and olive oil should be used to marinate and roast or grill mushroom caps until they are soft.

- Burgers should be assembled with red onion, tomato slices, red mushroom caps, spinach or arugula, and vegan mayo.

Vegan Thai Green Curry

Ingredients:

- One 14-ounce can of coconut milk

-2 tablespoons of green curry paste

- A variety of veggies, including carrots, bell peppers, and zucchini

- Cubed tofu, tempeh, or seitan

- Garnishing Thai basil leaves

- Jasmine rice, cooked

Preparation:

- Put coconut milk and green curry paste in a pot. Simmer for a while.

- Vegetables should be simmered with the tofu, tempeh, or seitan until they are soft.

- Serve with jasmine rice and garnish with Thai basil leaves.

Vegan Mediterranean Quinoa Salad

  Ingredients:

  - 2 cups cooked quinoa

- 1 sliced cucumber

- 1 diced tomato

  - 1/2 red onion, minced

- sliced Kalamata olives

  - Rinsed and drained chickpeas

  - Chopped fresh parsley

- Dressing of lemon juice and olive oil

  - To taste, salt and pepper

  Preparation:

  - Combine cooked quinoa with chickpeas, cucumber, tomato, red onion, and olives.

  - Dress with a dressing of lemon juice and olive oil.

  - Add fresh parsley, salt, and pepper to taste.

Vegan tofu and vegetable kebabs

  Ingredients:

- Cubed firm tofu

  - A variety of veggies, such as cherry tomatoes, bell peppers, zucchini, and red onions

  - Marinate (for example, with soy sauce, garlic, ginger, and olive oil)

  - Water-soaked wooden skewers

  Preparation:

- Skewers with tofu and vegetables should be used.

- Brush with marinade and cook vegetables and tofu until crisp.

Vegan Ratatouille
  Ingredients:
  - 1 sliced eggplant
- 1 sliced zucchini
- 1 sliced yellow squash
- 1 sliced red bell pepper
- 1 sliced onion
- 2 minced garlic cloves
- 1 can (14 oz) chopped up tomatoes
- Fresh rosemary and thyme
- Oil of olives
  - To taste, salt and pepper
  Preparation:
Vegetable slices are layered in a baking dish.
  - Combine olive oil, fresh herbs, garlic, crushed tomatoes, salt, and pepper.
  - When the vegetables are soft, pour the tomato mixture over them and bake.

Vegan Quesadillas with Black Beans and Corn
  Ingredients:
  - 8 small whole wheat tortillas
- 2 cups cooked and mashed black beans;
  - 1 cup of kernelized corn
  - 1 cup of shredded vegan cheese

- Guacamole and salsa for dipping

Preparation:

- Combine mashed black beans, corn, and vegan cheese on quesadillas.

- In a pan, cook the tortillas until they are crisp and the cheese is melted.

- Serve with guacamole and salsa for dipping.

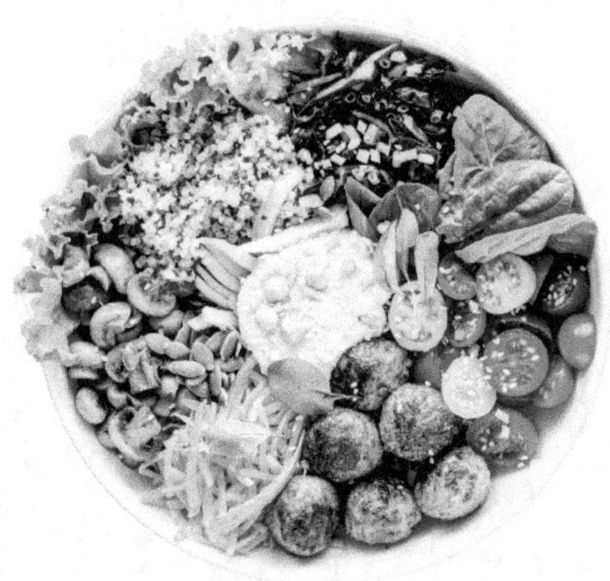

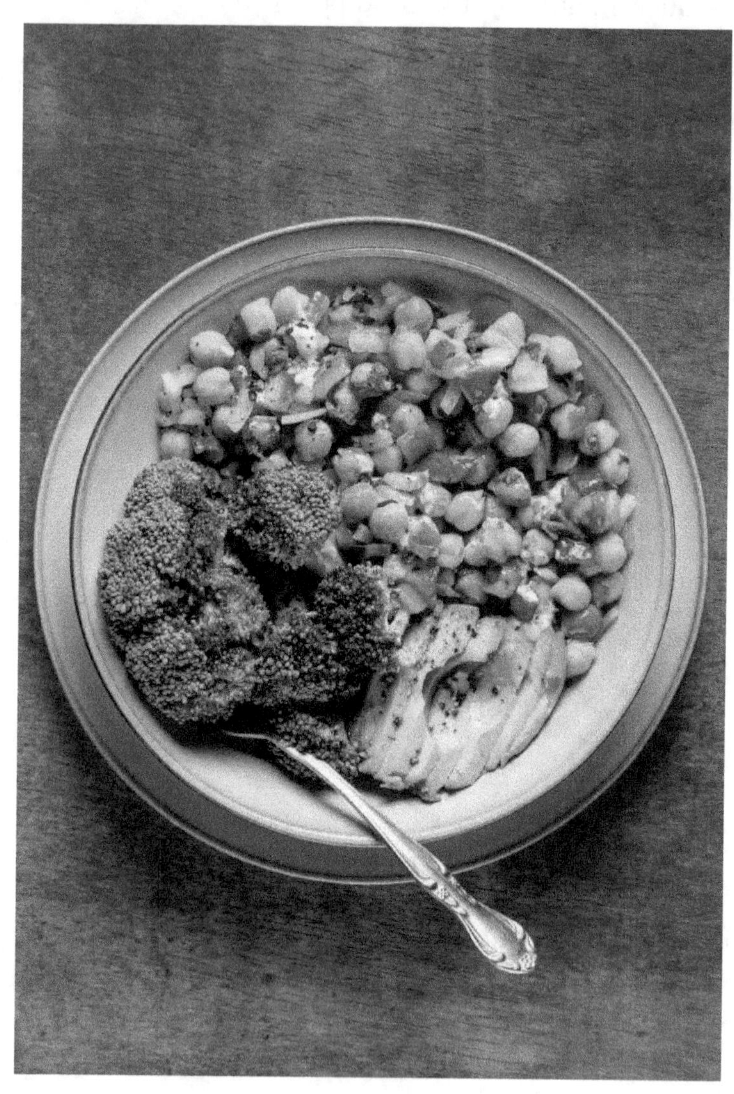

CHAPTER:6

Vegan pasta and Noodles

Traditional vegan aglio e olio spaghetti
Ingredients:
- 8 ounces of spaghetti
- 4 thinly sliced garlic cloves,
- 1/4 cup extra virgin olive oil,
- Salt, and black pepper to taste.
- Fresh parsley chopped finely for garnish

Instructions:
1. Prepare pasta as directed on the package. Drain, then set apart.
2. Heat the olive oil in a skillet, then add the garlic and red pepper flakes and cook until fragrant.
3. Combine the garlic oil mixture with the cooked pasta. Add salt and black pepper to taste.
4. Add chopped parsley as a garnish and serve.

Pasta with vegan pesto
Ingredients:
- 8 oz. of pasta (such as linguine or fettuccine)
- 2-cups of fresh basil leaves
- 1/4 cup nutritional yeast
- 1/2 cup pine nuts
- 2 garlic cloves

- Olive oil, 1/4 cup
- Pepper and salt, to taste
- Cherry tomatoes, if desired

Preparation:

1. Follow the directions on the pasta package to cook it. Drain, then set apart.

2. Combine basil, pine nuts, nutritional yeast, garlic, and olive oil in a food processor. Until smooth, blend.

3. Combine the pesto sauce with the cooked pasta. Add salt and pepper to taste.

4. If wanted, add cherry tomatoes and serve.

Alfredo pasta that is vegan

Ingredients:

- 8 ounces of fettuccine or linguine
- 1 cup soaked cashews (at least 4 hours)
- 1 cup of unsweetened almond milk
- 3 garlic cloves
- Nutritional yeast, 1/4 cup
- One lemon's juice
- Pepper and salt, to taste
- Garnishing with fresh parsley

Preparation:

1. Follow the directions on the pasta package to cook it. Drain, then set apart.

2. Blend soaked cashews, almond milk, nutritional yeast, garlic, lemon juice, salt, and pepper in a blender. until creamy, blend.

3. Combine the Alfredo sauce with the cooked pasta.

4. Add fresh parsley as a garnish and serve.

Vegan Macaroni & Cheese with Butternut Squash

Ingredients:

- 1 cup unsweetened almond milk
- 2 cups cubed butternut squash, and 8 ounces of macaroni.
- Nutritional yeast, 1/4 cup
- One-fourth cup vegan butter
- 1 teaspoon of garlic powder
- Pepper and salt, to taste
- Optional bread crumbs for topping

Instructions:

1. Prepare macaroni as directed on the packet. Drain, then set apart.

2. To make butternut squash soft, steam or bake it.

3. Put the cooked butternut squash, almond milk, nutritional yeast, vegan butter, garlic powder, salt, and pepper in a blender. Until smooth, blend.

4. Combine the cooked macaroni with the butternut squash sauce.

5. You can optionally sprinkle bread crumbs on top and bake until golden.

Vegan Thai Peanut Noodles

Ingredients:

- 8 ounces of rice noodles

- 1 tablespoon creamy peanut butter
-2 tablespoons soy sauce
-2 tablespoons lime juice
1-tablespoon maple syrup
- 1 teaspoon grated ginger
- 2 cloves minced garlic
- To taste, red pepper flakes
- Garnish with chopped cilantro and peanuts

Instructions:

1. Follow the package instructions when preparing rice noodles. Drain, and then separate.

2. Combine the peanut butter, soy sauce, maple syrup, lime juice, ginger, garlic, and red pepper flakes in a bowl.

3. Combine the peanut sauce with the cooked rice noodles.

4. Garnish with chopped cilantro and peanuts, before serving

Vegan mushroom stroganoff

Ingredients:

- 2 cups sliced mushrooms
- 8 ounces eggless pasta.
- 1 chopped onion
- 2 minced garlic cloves
- One cup of vegetable broth
- One cup of cashew cream (made by blending soaked cashews with water)

- 2-tablespoons of nutritional yeast
- 2 teaspoons soy sauce
- Add fresh parsley as garnish
- Add salt and pepper to taste

Instructions:

1. Prepare eggless pasta as directed on the packet. Drain, then set apart.

2. Saute mushrooms, onion, and garlic in a pan until they are soft.

3. Add the nutritional yeast, soy sauce, cashew cream, and vegetable broth. Stir and boil for a few minutes.

4. Add salt and pepper to taste.

5. Combine the stroganoff sauce and cooked noodles.

6. Add fresh parsley as a garnish and serve.

Vegan Zucchini Noodles with Pesto

Ingredients:

- 2 large spiralized zucchini
- 1 cup halved cherry tomatoes
- 1/2 cup vegan pesto (homemade or from a shop).
- Pine nuts as decoration
- Pepper and salt, to taste

Instructions:

1. Create zucchini noodles using a spiralizer.

2. Combine the cherry tomatoes and zucchini noodles in a big basin.

3. Add vegan pesto and toss.

4. Add salt and pepper to taste.

5. Before serving, garnish with pine nuts.

Vegan Ramen Noodle Soup
Ingredients:
- 8 ounces of ramen noodles
- 4 cups of veggie broth
- 2 chopped garlic cloves
- A cut, one-inch piece of ginger
- 2 cups of mixed vegetables (such as carrots, bok choy, and mushrooms)
- 2 tablespoons of soy sauce
2-tablespoon miso paste
- Tofu cubes as a garnish
- Garnishing green onions
Instructions:
1. Prepare the ramen noodles as directed on the package. Drain, then set apart.
2. Sauté the garlic and ginger until aromatic in a big pot.
3. Include veggie broth and simmer.
4. Once the miso paste has dissolved, add the soy sauce.
5. Include cubes of tofu and assorted vegetables. Cook the vegetables until they are soft.
6. Spoon the broth over the cooked ramen noodles in bowls.
7. Add green onions as a garnish and serve.

Vegetarian Lasagna with Spinach and Mushrooms
Ingredients:
- 12 lasagna noodles, prepared as directed on the package.
- Two cups of fresh spinach and two cups of chopped mushrooms
- 1 chopped onion
- 3 minced garlic cloves
- 2 cups vegan cheese
- Two cups of marinara sauce
- A serving of vegan mozzarella cheese
- Pepper and salt, to taste

Preparation:
1. In a pan, cook the mushrooms, onion, and garlic until they are soft.
2. Set the oven temperature to 375°F (190°C).
3. Place cooked lasagna noodles, sautéed mushrooms, fresh spinach, vegan ricotta, and marinara sauce in a baking dish.
4. Continue layering the ingredients until all are utilized, and then top with a layer of marinara sauce.
5. Add a sprinkle of vegan mozzarella cheese.
6. Bake for 25 minutes while covered with foil. Bake for an additional 10 minutes, or until bubbling and golden, after removing the foil.
7. Permit to slightly cool before serving.

Pad Thai vegan
Food ingredients:
- rice noodles in 8 oz.
-2 tablespoons vegetable oil
- 1 cup cubed tofu
- 1/2 cup chopped peanuts
- 1 cup bean sprouts
- 2 minced garlic cloves
- 2 chopped green onions
- Wedges of lime as a garnish
To the sauce:
- 1 tbsp maple syrup - 3 tbsp soy sauce - 2 tbsp tamarind
paste - 1 tsp sriracha sauce (adjust to taste)
Preparation:
1. Follow the package instructions for preparing the rice
noodles. Drain, and then separate.
2. Combine all the sauce ingredients in a small bowl.
3. Sauté tofu in hot vegetable oil in a big skillet until it
becomes crispy.
4. Quickly sauté the green onions and minced garlic in
the skillet.
5. Include the prepared sauce and cooked rice noodles in
the skillet. Combine by tossing.
6. Arrange bean sprouts, chopped peanuts, and lime
wedges on top to serve.

Pasta with vegan lemon asparagus.

Ingredients:

- 1 bunch of trimmed and diced asparagus

- 8 ounces of spaghetti.

- One lemon's juice and zest

- 2 minced garlic cloves

- To taste, add red pepper flakes to 1/4 cup of olive oil.

- Black pepper and salt, to taste

- Garnish: fresh basil leaves

Preparation:

1. First, prepare the spaghetti according to the directions on the package. Drain, then set apart.

2. Sauté asparagus in hot olive oil until fork-tender.

3. Include the minced garlic, red pepper flakes, salt, black pepper, lemon zest, and lemon juice. For one minute, sauté.

4. Add the lemon asparagus sauce to the cooked spaghetti.

5. Add fresh basil leaves as a garnish and serve.

Pasta with Roasted Red Peppers that is vegan.

Ingredients:

- 8 oz. penne pasta

- Two large red bell peppers that have been roasted and skinned

- Half a cup of raw cashews that have been soaked for at least four hours.

- 2 minced garlic cloves

- Nutritional yeast, 1/4 cup
- 1/4 cup veggie broth
- Black pepper and salt (to taste)
- Garnish of fresh basil

Instructions:

1. Make the penne pasta according to the directions on the package. Drain, and then separate.

2. Blend roasted red peppers, soaked cashews, nutritional yeast, minced garlic, vegetable broth, salt, and black pepper in a blender. until creamy, blend.

3. Combine the roasted red pepper sauce with the cooked penne pasta.

4. Before serving, garnish with fresh basil.

Vegan Cilantro Lime Pasta

Ingredients:

- 1 cup of fresh cilantro leaves
- 8 ounces of linguine
- 14 cup cashews
- Two limes' juice
- 2 minced garlic cloves
- Olive oil, 1/4 cup
- Black pepper and salt, to taste
- Cherry tomatoes, sliced as a garnish

Instructions:

1. Prepare the linguine as directed on the packet. Drain, then set apart.

2. Combine cilantro, cashews, lime juice, chopped garlic, olive oil, salt, and black pepper in a food processor. Until smooth, blend.

3. Combine the cilantro lime sauce with the cooked linguine.

4. Add sliced cherry tomatoes as a garnish before serving.

Sweet potato noodles made vegan with a creamy cashew sauce

Ingredients:

- Two medium sweet potatoes, spiralized to make noodles.

- 1/2 cup cashews (soaked for at least 4 hours)

- 1 cup cherry tomatoes, cut in half.

- Nutritional yeast, 1/4 cup

- 2 garlic cloves

1/4 cup of water

- Pepper and salt, to taste

- Garnish of fresh basil

Instructions:

1. Make sweet potato noodles by spiralizing them.

2. Put soaked cashews, nutritional yeast, garlic, water, salt, and pepper in a blender. until creamy, blend.

3. In a pan, cook sweet potato noodles until they are soft.

4. Combine the creamy cashew sauce with the cooked sweet potato noodles.

5. Add fresh basil as a garnish and serve.

Vegan Pumpkin Sage Pasta
Ingredients:
- 8 oz. of fettuccine,
- 1 cup of pumpkin puree
- 1/2 cup of coconut milk
- Nutritional yeast, 1/4 cup
- 1-teaspoon dried sage
- 2 minced garlic cloves
- Black pepper and salt, to taste
- Fresh sage chopped finely for garnish

Instructions:
1. Prepare the fettuccine as directed on the package. Drain, then set apart.
2. Put pumpkin puree, coconut milk, nutritional yeast, sage, minced garlic, salt, and pepper in a pot. For a few minutes, simmer.
3. Add the pumpkin sage sauce to the cooked fettuccine.
4. Before serving, garnish with finely chopped fresh sage.

Vegan Broccoli Pesto Pasta
Ingredients:
- 2 cups of cooked broccoli florets
- 8 ounces of penne pasta.
- 1-cup of fresh basil leaves
- Almonds, 1/2 cup
- 2 garlic cloves
- Olive oil, 1/4 cup

- Lemon juice, as desired
- Black pepper and salt, to taste
- Garnish: vegan Parmesan cheese

Instructions:

1. Make the penne pasta according to the directions on the package. Drain, and then separate.

2. Place steamed broccoli, basil leaves, almonds, garlic, olive oil, lemon juice, salt, and black pepper in a food processor. Until smooth, blend.

3. Combine the broccoli pesto with the cooked penne pasta.

4. Before serving, garnish with vegan Parmesan cheese.

Vegan Sun-Dried Tomato and Spinach Pasta

Ingredients:

- 8 oz. rotini pasta
- 1/2 cup. sun-dried tomatoes-sliced, rehydrated, and dried tomatoes
- 2 cups of fresh spinach
- 2 minced garlic cloves
- Pine nuts, 1/4 cup
- Olive oil, 1/4 cup
- Black pepper and salt, to taste
- Garnishment of lemon zest

Instructions:

1. Prepare the rotini pasta as directed on the packet. Drain, then set apart.

2. Sauté minced garlic in a skillet until fragrant.

3. Include new spinach and rehydrated sun-dried tomatoes. Sauté spinach till it wilts.

4. Combine the sun-dried tomato and spinach combination with the cooked rotini pasta.

5. Toast pine nuts until they are golden in a separate pan.

6. Before serving, sprinkle some toasted pine nuts and lemon zest on top of the pasta.

Vegan Mediterranean Pasta Salad
Ingredients:
- Fusilli pasta
- 8 ounces
- 1 cup chopped cherry tomatoes
- 1 cup diced cucumber
- 1/2 cup pitted and sliced Kalamata olives
- 1/4 cup finely chopped red onion
- 1/4 cup chopped fresh parsley
- 1/4 cup olive oil.
- 1 teaspoon dried oregano
- 2 tablespoon balsamic vinegar
- Black pepper and salt, to taste

Instructions:
1. Prepare the fusilli pasta as directed on the packet. Drain, then set apart.

2. Combine cherry tomatoes, cucumber, and Kalamata olives in a sizable bowl. red onion, olives, and fresh parsley.

3. Combine olive oil, balsamic vinegar, dried oregano, salt, and black pepper in a small bowl.

4. Combine the cooked fusilli pasta with the vinaigrette and the Mediterranean salad ingredients.

5. Before serving, chill in the fridge.

Vegan Spicy Soba Noodles
Ingredients:
- 8 ounces of soba noodles
- 2 tablespoons of sesame oil
- 2 chopped garlic cloves
- 1 inch of grated ginger
- 2 tablespoons of soy sauce
- One tablespoon of Sriracha sauce, to taste
- 2 cups stirred together-fry veggies (such as carrots, bell peppers, and snow peas) - top with green onions and sesame seeds

Instructions:
1. Prepare soba noodles as directed on the package. Drain, then set apart.

2. Heat sesame oil in a wok or sizable pan, then add the minced garlic and grated ginger. Cook until fragrant.

3. Stir in the sriracha sauce and soy sauce to the skillet.

4. Add the various stir-fry vegetables and simmer for 4 minutes or until cooked.

5. Combine the hot stir-fry mixture with the cooked soba noodles.

6. Before serving, garnish with sesame seeds and thinly sliced green onions.

Baked pasta with spinach and artichokes that is vegan
Ingredients:
- 8 ounces of penne pasta
- 1 cup of chopped spinach
- 1 can of chopped, drained artichoke hearts
- A serving of vegan cream cheese
- One-fourth cup vegan mayonnaise
Nutritional yeast, 1/4 cup
- 2 minced garlic cloves
- Black pepper and salt, to taste
- Topping of vegan mozzarella cheese
Preparation:
1. Prepare the penne pasta in accordance with the directions on the package. Drain, then set apart.
2. Set the oven temperature to 375°F (190°C).
3. Combine chopped spinach, chopped artichoke hearts, vegan mayonnaise, nutritional yeast, minced garlic, salt, and pepper in a sizable bowl.
4. Stir the cooked penne pasta into the bowl.
5. Place vegan mozzarella cheese on top of the mixture in a baking tray.
6. Bake the dish for 20 to 25 minutes, or until the cheese is bubbling and melted.
7. Permit to slightly cool before serving.

CHAPTER:7

Sides And Accompaniment

Roasted Garlic Hummus

Ingredients:

- 2 cans of rinsed and drained chickpeas
- 4 cloves of roasted garlic.
- 1 lemon juice
- 3 tablespoons of olive oil
- 2 teaspoons of tahini
- Put salt and pepper to taste

Preparation:

1. Place everything in a food processor and process until smooth.

2. Modify the seasoning as necessary. Serve with vegetables or pita bread.

Sweet Potatoes, Mashed

Ingredients:

- Three large sweet potatoes that have been peeled and diced
- Two tablespoons of vegan butter
- One-fourth cup of almond milk.
  - Add salt and pepper to taste

Make:

1. Boil sweet potatoes until they are fork-tender, then drain.

2. Blend till smooth using almond milk and vegan butter.

3. Salt and pepper to taste.

Quinoa Salad

Ingredients:
- 1 cup cooked and cooled quinoa
- 1 cup diced cucumber
- 1 cup diced tomatoes
- 1/2 cup chopped fresh parsley
- 1/4 cup finely chopped red onion
- 1 lemon's juice
- 2 tablespoons of extra virgin olive oil.
- To taste ,add salt and pepper

Make:

1. In a big basin, mix together all the ingredients.
2. Thoroughly combine and chill before serving.

Asparagus That Has Been Grill

Ingredients:
- 1 bunch trimmed asparagus
- Olive oil, 2 tablespoons
- Put Salt and pepper to taste

Prepare:

1. Season the asparagus with salt, pepper, and olive oil.

2. Grill the food for 3 to 5 minutes, or until it's soft and barely browned.

Buffalo Bites with Cauliflower

Ingredients Include :

- one head of cauliflower that has been sliced into florets
- Half a cup of buffalo sauce
- One tablespoon of olive oil.

Setting up:

1. Roast cauliflower for 20 minutes at 400°F (200°C) after tossing with olive oil.

2. After taking the dish out of the oven, drizzle it with buffalo sauce and bake it for another 10 minutes.

Garlic and Sautéed Spinach

Ingredients:

- 1 pound of fresh spinach
- 2 minced garlic cloves.
- Olive oil, 1 tbsp
- Put salt and pepper to taste

Preparation:

1. Add garlic to a skillet of hot olive oil and cook until fragrant.

2. After adding, boil spinach until it wilts. Add salt and pepper to taste.

Vegetarian coleslaw

Ingredients:

- 4 cups of finely chopped cabbage and carrots
- Half a cup vegan mayo
- 1 tablespoon Dijon mustard
- 2 teaspoons apple cider vinegar
- 1 tablespoon maple syrup
- Salt and pepper to taste

Instructions:

1. Combine the cabbage and carrots in a big basin.

2. Combine vegan mayonnaise, vinegar, mustard, and maple syrup in another bowl.

3. Drizzle the vegetables with the dressing and toss to coat. Add salt and pepper to taste.

Bell Peppers Stuffed

Ingredients:

- 1 cup cooked quinoa
- 1 cup cooked and drained black beans
- 1 cup corn kernels
- 4 bell peppers with tops and seeds removed.
- 1 cup tomatoes, diced
- 1 teaspoon chili powder
- 1/2 cup diced red onion
- To taste, salt and pepper

Setting up:

1. In a bowl, combine the following ingredients: quinoa, black beans, corn, tomatoes, red onion, chili powder, salt, and pepper.

2. Stuff the bell peppers with the mixture and bake for 25 to 30 minutes at 375°F (190°C).

Roasted Beet Salad

Ingredients:
- 2 tablespoons each of olive oil
- balsamic vinegar
- 1/4 cup chopped fresh basil
- 4 medium beets, peeled and diced.
- To taste, salt and pepper

Setting up:

1. Combine olive oil, salt, and pepper with the beets.
2. Roast for 30 to 35 minutes at 400 °F (200 °C).
3. Drizzle balsamic vinegar over the dish and add fresh basil as a garnish.

Crisp Baked Zucchini Fries

Ingredients:
- Two zucchini, sliced into fries.
- Panko breadcrumbs, 1 cup
- 1 teaspoon of garlic powder
- 1/2 cup of nutritional yeast
- Put salt and pepper to taste

Preparation:

1. Set the oven temperature to 425°F (220°C).

2. Combine nutritional yeast, panko breadcrumbs, garlic powder, salt, and pepper in a bowl.

3. Spread the breadcrumb mixture over the zucchini fries and bake for 20 to 25 minutes.

Roasted Brussels sprouts with garlic
Ingredients:
- 1 pound chopped and half Brussels sprouts
- 3 minced garlic cloves.
- Olive oil, 2 tablespoons
- Add salt and pepper to taste

Make:

1. Combine olive oil, garlic, salt, and pepper with the Brussels sprouts.

2. Roast for 25 to 30 minutes at 400 °F (200 °C).

Baba Ganoush
Ingredients:
- Two large eggplants.
- 3 minced garlic cloves
- 2 tablespoons tahini
- 1 lemon's juice
- Olive oil, 2 tablespoons
- Add salt and pepper to taste

Preparation:

1. After roasting eggplants until the flesh is soft, remove the flesh.

2. Combine the garlic, tahini, lemon juice, olive oil, salt, and pepper with the eggplant meat.

Cucumber Dill Salad

Ingredients:

1 tablespoon olive oil

2 thinly sliced cucumbers

1/4 cup chopped fresh dill

2 tablespoons white vinegar.

Prepare:

Toss cucumbers with dill, vinegar, olive oil, salt, and pepper in a bowl. Season with salt and pepper to taste.

Vegetarian Garlic Bread

Substances:

- 1 sliced baguette
- 1/2 cup vegan butter
- minced 4 cloves of garlic
- 2 teaspoons freshly chopped parsley

Setting up:

1. Combine vegan butter, parsley, and minced garlic.

2. Spread the mixture on the baguette pieces and bake for 10 to 12 minutes at 350°F (175°C).

Pickled Carrots with Spice
   Ingredients:
- 1 pound of peeled and sliced carrots
- 2 tablespoons of olive oil
- 1 teaspoon of paprika.
  -Salt and pepper to taste
- Half teaspoon of cayenne pepper
   Setting up:

1. Combine olive oil, paprika, cayenne, salt, and pepper with the carrots.

2. Roast for 20 to 25 minutes at 425 °F (220 °C).

Potato salad that is vegan
   Ingredients:
- 3 pounds of diced, boiling potatoes
- 1/2 cup vegan mayo
- 2 teaspoons Dijon mustard
- 1/4 cup fresh dill that has been minced,
- 1/4 cup sliced red onion.
- Add salt and pepper to taste
 Make:

1. In a bowl, mix together the potatoes, vegan mayonnaise, Dijon mustard, dill, red onion, salt, and pepper.

Broccoli With Lemon Roasting
Ingredients:
   - 1 pound of broccoli florets

-   Olive oil, 2 tablespoons

 - One lemon's juice and zest

 - Put salt and pepper to taste

Make:

1. Toss the broccoli with the olive oil, lemon juice, zest, and seasonings.

2. Roast for 20 to 25 minutes at 425 °F (220 °C).

Stuffed mushrooms

Ingredients:

- 16 big mushrooms cut after the stems have been removed

1/2 cup breadcrumbs.

- 2 minced garlic cloves

 - 1/4 cup vegan cream cheese

- 2 teaspoons freshly chopped parsley

- Salt and pepper to taste

Preparation:

1. Combine breadcrumbs, vegan cream cheese, garlic, parsley, salt, and pepper with chopped mushroom stems.

2. Fill the mushroom caps with the mixture and bake for 20 minutes at 375°F (190°C).

Soup with lentils and vegetables

Ingredients:

- 1 cup dry, rinsed, and drained green or brown lentils

- 4 cups of vegetable broth

- 2 diced carrots

- 2 chopped celery stalks

- 1 diced onion

- 2 minced garlic cloves

1 tsp. dried thyme

- To taste, salt and pepper

Setting up:

1. In a big pot, soften the celery, carrots, onion, and garlic.

2. Include the vegetable broth, thyme, lentils, salt, and pepper.

3. Simmer until lentils are soft, about 30 to 40 minutes.

Veggie Sushi Rolls

Ingredients:

- 2 cups of cooked sushi rice that has been seasoned with rice vinegar and 10 sheets of nori (seaweed).

- Thinly sliced veggies, including carrot, bell pepper, avocado, and cucumber;

- Soy sauce and wasabi for dipping

Setting up:

1. Spread a clean area with a bamboo sushi rolling mat.

2. Lay a sheet of nori on top of a sheet of plastic wrap on the mat.

3. Leaving a border, apply a thin coating of sushi rice on the nori.

4. Place thinly sliced vegetables in the middle.

5. Use the mat and plastic wrap to firmly roll the sushi, then cut into bite-sized pieces.

6. Add wasabi and soy sauce before serving.

Enjoy these delectable plant-based recipes for sides and accompaniments!

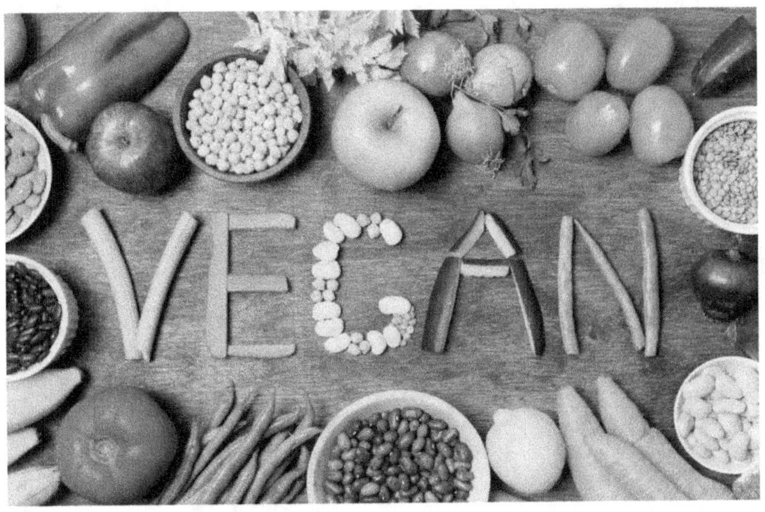

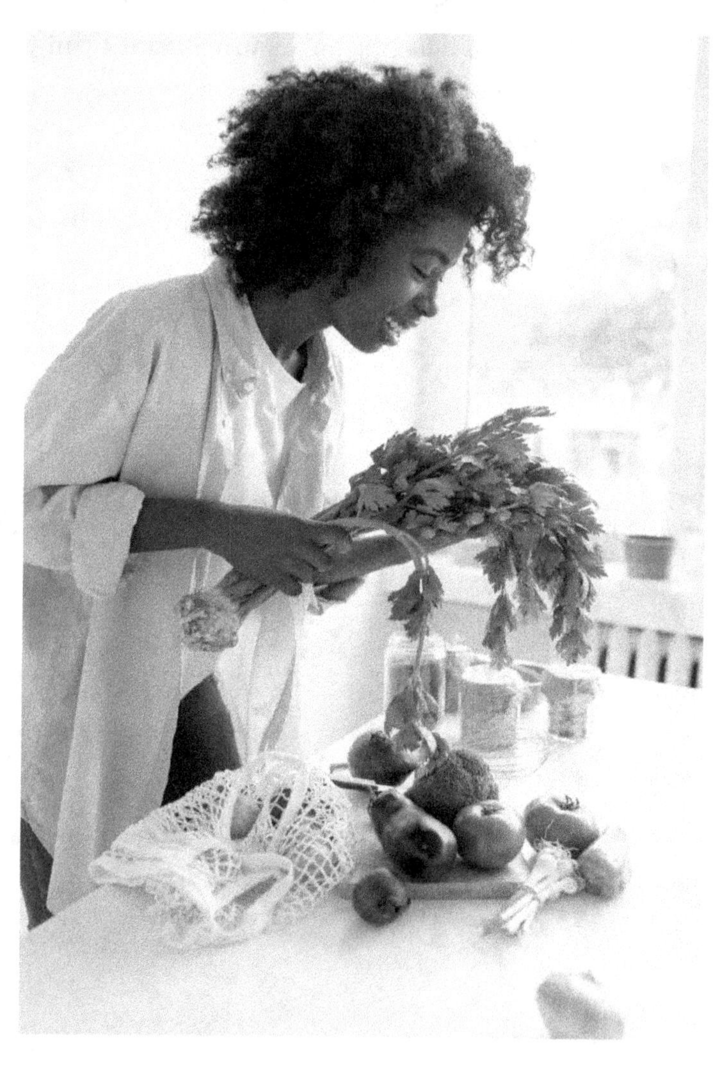

CHAPTER:8

Breads And Baked Goods

Vegan banana bread
  Ingredients:
- Three ripe bananas that have been mashed.
- One-fourth cup coconut oil
- A half cup of maple syrup
- 1 1/2 cups whole wheat flour
- 1 teaspoon vanilla extract
- 1 teaspoon baking soda
 - Half teaspoon of salt
- 1/2 cup chopped walnuts (optional)
  - **Setting up:**
   1. Set the oven's temperature to 350°F (175°C).

   2. Combine mashed bananas with coconut oil, maple syrup, vanilla, and a bowl.

   3. Combine flour, baking soda, and salt in another basin.

   4. Combine the wet and dry ingredients; if preferred, fold in the chopped walnuts.

   5. Place a greased loaf pan with the mixture in it, and bake for 55 to 60 minutes, or until a toothpick inserted into the center comes out clean.

Vegan whole-wheat pancakes
Ingredients:

- 1 cup whole wheat flour
- 1 tablespoon sugar
- 1 teaspoon baking powder.
- 0.5 teaspoon baking soda
- 1 cup almond milk (or any other plant-based milk)
- 1/4 teaspoon salt
- 1 teaspoon of vanilla extract
- 1 tablespoon of apple cider vinegar
- **Setting up:**

1. In a bowl, combine the almond milk and apple cider vinegar. Let the mixture sit for five minutes to curdle.

2. Combine the flour, sugar, baking soda, baking powder, and salt in a separate bowl.

3. Combine the dry ingredients with the almond milk mixture and vanilla essence.

4. Stir just until incorporated.

5. Pour 1/4 cup batter per pancake into a nonstick skillet that has been heated to medium-high heat. Cook until bubbles appear on the surface. Cook till golden brown after flipping.

Vegetarian Zucchini Bread
Ingredients:

1 cup unsweetened applesauce
2 cups grated zucchini

- 1/4 cup maple syrup
 - One-fourth cup coconut sugar
- Two teaspoons of vanilla essence
- Two cups of whole wheat flour, and one teaspoon of baking soda
- 1/2 teaspoon of baking powder
 - 1 teaspoon ground cinnamon
- Half teaspoon of salt

- Setting up:

1. Grease a loaf pan and set the oven to 350°F (175°C).

2. Combine the zucchini, applesauce, vanilla, maple syrup, and coconut sugar in a bowl.

3. Combine the flour, baking soda, baking powder, salt, and cinnamon in a separate bowl.

4. Combine the ingredients and pour the mixture onto the pan that has been prepared.

5. Bake for between 50 and 60 minutes, or until a toothpick is clean.

Veggie Blueberry Muffins

Ingredients:
- Two cups of all-purpose flour
- one tablespoon of baking powder,
- Half a cup of sugar.
- 1 cup almond milk (or any other plant-based milk)
- 1/2 teaspoon salt
- One-fourth cup coconut oil

- 1 teaspoon of vanilla extract

- Either fresh or frozen blueberries,1 ½ cups

- Setting up:

1. Line a muffin pan with liners and preheat the oven to 375°F (190°C).

2. Mix the flour, sugar, baking soda, and salt in a bowl.

3. Combine almond milk, coconut oil, and vanilla in a separate bowl.

4. Stir slightly to incorporate after adding the wet components to the dry ones. Add blueberries and fold.

5. Spoon the batter into the muffin tins, and bake for 20 to 25 minutes, or until a toothpick inserted in the center comes out clean.

Veggie cinnamon rolls

Ingredients for the Dough include:

- 1/4 cup coconut oil

- 1 cup almond milk (or any other plant-based milk)

- 1 packet (2 1/4 tsp) of active dry yeast

- 1/4 cup sugar

- 3 cups of all-purpose flour

- 1/2 teaspoon of salt

- Regarding the Filling

- 1/4 cup melted coconut oil

- 2 tablespoon of ground cinnamon

- Half cup of brown sugar

- To Add the Icing

- 1 cup of powdered sugar

- 2 tablespoons of almond milk

- 1/8 teaspoon of vanilla extract

- Setting up:

1. Warm up the coconut oil and almond milk without bringing them to a boil. Add sugar after removing from heat. Allow the yeast to rest on top of the mixture for ten minutes.

2. To the yeast mixture, add 3 cups of flour and some salt. After smoothing it out, cover it and let it rise for an hour.

3. Form the dough into a rectangle, brush it with melted coconut oil, and then top it with cinnamon and brown sugar.

4. Log the dough and cut it into rolls.

5. Put the rolls in a prepared pan and bake for 25 to 30 minutes at 350 °F (175 °C).

6. To make the frosting, combine powdered sugar, almond milk, and vanilla essence. Drizzle it over the warm rolls.

Vegan Garlic Herb Breadsticks

- Substances:

- 1 lb of store-bought pizza dough or homemade pizza dough

- 2 tablespoons of olive oil

- 2 chopped garlic cloves

- 1-teaspoon dried basil

-1 teaspoon of dried oregano

- 1/4 teaspoon black pepper

- 1/2 teaspoon salt

- **Setting up:**

1. Set the oven's temperature to 425°F (220°C).

2. On a floured board, roll out the pizza dough into a rectangle.

3. To make breadsticks, slice the dough into strips.

4. Position a baking sheet with the breadsticks on it.

5. In a small bowl, combine the olive oil, garlic, basil, oregano, salt, and black pepper. Apply a coat of this mixture to the breadsticks.

6. Bake until golden brown for 12 to 15 minutes.

Pumpkin Bread Made Vegan

Ingredients:

- whole wheat flour 1 3/4 cups

- Baking soda, 1 teaspoon

- 1/2 teaspoon of baking powder

- 1 teaspoon of ground cinnamon

- 1/2 tsp salt

- 1/8 teaspoon ground nutmeg

- 1/2 teaspoon crushed cloves

- One-fourth cup coconut oil

- A half cup of maple syrup

- 1 cup of pure can pumpkin

- 1/4 cup plant-based milk, such as almond milk

1 teaspoon vanilla essence

Preparation:

1. Grease a loaf pan and preheat the oven to 350°F (175°C).

2. Flour, baking soda, baking powder, salt, and spices should be combined in a bowl.

3. Combine coconut oil, maple syrup, pumpkin puree, almond milk, and vanilla in a separate bowl.

4. After combining the ingredients, pour the mixture into the prepared pan.

5. Bake for between 50 and 60 minutes, or until a toothpick is clean.

Cookies with chocolate chips made from plants

Ingredients:

- Melted 1/2 cup coconut oil
- 1/4 cup of granulated sugar
- 1/2 cup of brown sugar
- 1/4 cup plant-based milk, such as almond milk
- 1 teaspoon of vanilla extract
- Two cups of all-purpose flour
- one-half teaspoon of baking soda
- 1 cup dairy-free chocolate chips
- 1/2 tsp. salt

- Setting up:

1. Prepare a baking sheet with parchment paper, and preheat the oven to 350°F (175°C).

2. Combine melted coconut oil, brown sugar, sugar crystals, almond milk, and vanilla in a bowl.

3. Add flour, baking soda, and salt in a separate bowl.

4. After combining the dry and wet ingredients, mix in the chocolate chips.

5. Place dough spoonfuls on the baking sheet and bake for 10 to 12 minutes, or until the edges are golden brown.

Vegetarian Cornbread

Ingredients:

- 1 cup all-purpose flour
- 1 cup cornmeal
- 1/4 cup sugar
- 1 teaspoon baking powder.
- 1 cup almond milk (or any other plant-based milk)
- 1/2 teaspoon salt
- 1/4 cup melted coconut oil
- 1/4 cup applesauce

- Setting up:

1. Grease an 8 × 8-inch baking dish and preheat the oven to 425°F (220°C).

2. Add together the cornmeal, flour, sugar, baking soda, and salt in a bowl.

3. Combine almond milk, applesauce, and melted coconut oil in a separate bowl.

4. Stir slightly to incorporate after adding the wet components to the dry ones.

5. Place the baking dish in the oven and bake the batter for 20 to 25 minutes, or until golden brown.

Pumpkin Muffins Made From Plants

Ingredients:

- 1.5 cups whole wheat flour
- 1 teaspoon baking soda.
- 1/2 teaspoon of baking powder
- 1/2 teaspoon salt
- 1 teaspoon cinnamon, ground
- 1/8 teaspoon ground nutmeg
- 1/4 teaspoon of powdered cloves
- 1 cup of pure can pumpkin
- 1/4 cup of maple syrup
- Half cup of coconut sugar
- 1/4 cup melted coconut oil
- 1/4 cup almond milk (or any other plant-based milk)
- 1 teaspoon of vanilla extract

- Setting up:

1. Line a muffin pan with liners and preheat the oven to 350°F (175°C).

2. Combine the flour, baking soda, baking powder, salt, and spices in a basin.

3. Combine pumpkin puree, melted coconut oil, maple syrup, almond milk, and vanilla in a separate bowl.

4. After combining the dry and wet ingredients, divide the batter among the muffin tins.

5. Bake for 20 to 25 minutes, or until a toothpick is clean.

Veggie Focaccia with Herbs

Ingredients:

- 1 lb pizza dough, either homemade or purchased.
- 2 tablespoons of olive oil
- 2 chopped garlic cloves
- 1 teaspoon of dried rosemary
- 1-teaspoon dried thyme
- 1/4 teaspoon of black pepper
- 1/2 teaspoon of salt

- Setting up:

1. Set oven temperature to 425°F (220°C).

2. On a floured board, roll out the pizza dough into a rectangle or a circle.

3. Place a baking sheet with the dough on it.

4. In a bowl, combine olive oil, chopped garlic, dried thyme, dried rosemary, salt, and black pepper.

5. Spread the dough with the oil mixture.

6. Make divots in the dough with your fingertips.

7. Bake until golden brown, about 20 to 25 minutes.

Pumpkin Pie Made From Plants

For the Crust: - Ingredients

- Use vegan Graham crackers to make 1 1/4 cups of crumbs.
- 1/4 cup coconut oil that has melted

- Regarding the Filling:

- 1 15-ounce can of pureed pumpkin
- 3/4 cup full-fat coconut milk

- Half a cup of brown sugar
 - 1 teaspoon cinnamon
 - 1/4 cup cornstarch
- 1/8 teaspoon ground nutmeg
- 1/4 teaspoon of powdered cloves
- Salt, 1/4 teaspoon
- **For the Optional Topping:**
- Whipped coconut cream
   - **Setting up:**
    1. Set oven temperature to 350°F (175°C).
    2. Combine melted coconut oil and graham cracker crumbs. To create the crust, press this mixture into a pie pan.
    3. Blend pumpkin puree, coconut milk, brown sugar, cornstarch, spices, and salt to a creamy consistency in a blender.
    4. Fill the crust with the contents.
    5. Bake the filling until it is set, about 50 to 60 minutes.
    6. Before serving, allow it to cool, and if preferred, top with coconut whipped cream.

Vegan lemon poppy seed muffins
Ingredients:
- Two cups of all-purpose flour
- one tablespoon of baking powder
- Half a cup of sugar.
- 0.5 teaspoon baking soda

- 1/2 teaspoon salt
- 1/4 cup coconut oil that has melted
- 1 cup plant-based milk (such as almond milk)
- 1/4 cup lemon juice
 - 2 lemons' zest
- A teaspoon of vanilla extract
- Two tablespoons of poppy seeds
   - Setting up:
1. Line a muffin pan with liners and preheat the oven to 375°F (190°C).

2. Combine the flour, sugar, baking soda, baking powder, and salt in a basin.

3. Combine melted coconut oil, almond milk, lemon juice, lemon zest, and vanilla in a separate bowl.

4. After combining the dry and wet ingredients, fold in the poppy seeds.

5. Spoon the batter into the muffin tins, and bake for 18 to 20 minutes, or until a toothpick inserted in the center comes out clean.

Scones made of plants

Ingredients:
- Two cups of all-purpose flour
- one-fourth cup of sugar
- 1-tablespoon baking powder
- 1/2 teaspoon salt
- 1/2 cup cold vegan butter (crumbled)
- 1 cup plant-based almond milk

- 1 teaspoon of vanilla extract
- 1/2 cup of optional dried fruit or chocolate chips
  - **Setting up:**

1. Prepare a baking sheet with parchment paper, and preheat the oven to 425°F (220°C).

2. Mix the flour, sugar, baking soda, and salt in a bowl.

3. Add the cold vegan butter and mix it into the flour with a pastry cutter or your fingers until you have coarse crumbs.

4. Combine vanilla essence and almond milk before adding to the dry ingredients.

5. If preferred, fold in chocolate chips or dried fruit.

6. Roll the dough out onto a floured surface, cut it into eight wedges, and form a circle out of it.

7. Spread the scones out on a baking sheet, and bake for 12 to 15 minutes, or until golden brown.

Vegan chocolate zucchini bread

Ingredients:
- 1 1/2 cups shredded zucchini
- 1/2 cup unsweetened applesauce
- 1/4 cup melted coconut oil
 - A half cup of maple syrup
 - 1 teaspoon of vanilla extract
- 1/2 cup chocolate powder
- 1 1/2 cups whole wheat flour
- 1 teaspoon baking soda

- 1/2 teaspoon of baking powder
- 1/2 teaspoon salt
- Half a cup of dairy chocolate chips that aren't.
  - Setting up:

1. Grease a loaf pan and set the oven to 350°F (175°C).

2. Combine grated zucchini, applesauce, maple syrup, vanilla, and melted coconut oil in a bowl.

3. Combine flour, cocoa powder, baking soda, baking powder, and salt in a separate basin.

4. After combining the dry and wet ingredients, mix in the chocolate chips.

5. Spoon the mixture into the prepared pan, and bake for 50 to 60 minutes, or until a toothpick inserted in the center comes out clean.

CHAPTER:9

Gluten Free Procedures

Quinoa Salad with Roasted Vegetables,
 Ingredients include:

- 1 cup of quinoa
- A variety of veggies such as bell peppers, zucchini, and carrots.
- Oil of olives
 - Pepper and salt
   - Setting up:
   1. Prepare the quinoa as directed on the packaging.
   2. Toss chopped vegetables with salt, pepper, and olive oil before roasting until soft.
   3. Combine the cooked quinoa with the roasted vegetables, top with your preferred dressing, and serve.

Chickpea and Spinach Curry
 Ingredients:

- 2 cans rinsed and drained chickpeas
- 1 chopped onion
- 2 minced garlic cloves
- 1 can of chopped tomatoes
 2 cups of spinach
- 1 teaspoon curry powder
- Salt and pepper to taste

-**Make**:

1. Sauté the garlic and onion until aromatic.

2. Include curry powder, tomatoes, and chickpeas. Cook for ten minutes.

3. Add spinach and stir until wilted. Add salt and pepper to taste.

Pesto-topped Zucchini Noodles:
Ingredients:
- Three to four medium zucchini and a cup of fresh basil leaves
- Two garlic cloves
- 1/4 cup of pine nuts
- Olive oil, 1/4 cup
- Nutritional yeast and salt, if desired
- **Setting up:**
1. Use spiralizer when making zucchini noodles.
2. To prepare pesto, combine basil, pine nuts, garlic, and olive oil.

3. Add nutritional yeast and salt to the tossed zucchini noodles before tossing with pesto.

Sweet Potato and Black Bean Tacos:
- **Ingredients:**
- 1 can of washed and drained black beans
- 2 large sweet potatoes
- 1 teaspoon of chili powder
- Tacos made of corn

- Your choice of toppings (lettuce, avocado, salsa)
  - **Setting up:**
    1. Sweet potato cubes are roasted with chili powder until they are soft.
    2. Warm up black beans.
    3. Add your preferred toppings to corn tortillas along with sweet potatoes and black beans.

Stuffed bell peppers with mushrooms and spinach:
  Ingredients:
- 4 halved bell peppers with seeds removed
- 2 cups chopped mushrooms
- 2 cups spinach
- 1 diced onion
- 2 minced garlic cloves
-1 tomato dice from a can
 - Put salt and pepper to taste
- **Make:**
    1. Soften the onion and garlic in a skillet.
 2. Add the mushrooms and sauté them until the moisture is released.
    3. Add the spinach and tomato dice. Cook spinach until it wilts.
    4. Insert the mushroom and spinach mixture into the bell pepper halves. Bake peppers until they are soft.

Stir-fried vegetables and lentils:
   Ingredients:
- Assorted stir-fry vegetables, such as broccoli, bell peppers, and snap peas
- 1 cup cooked dry green lentils
- 2 tablespoons of gluten-free soy sauce
- 1-tablespoon sesame oil
- 1 teaspoon minced ginger
- 2 minced garlic cloves
   - Setting up:
1. In sesame oil, stir-fry veggies until they are crisp-tender.

2. Add soy sauce, ginger, garlic, and cooked lentils. Cook until well heated for a few minutes.

Cauliflower pizza crust:
Ingredients:
- 1 head of grated cauliflower
- 2 flax eggs (2 tbsp powdered flaxseed and 6 tbsp water).
- Half a cup of almond meal
- 1 teaspoon of dried oregano
- Salt and pepper to taste
Make:
1. Steam the cauliflower, then press off any extra moisture.

2. To produce a dough, combine cauliflower, flax eggs, almond meal, oregano, salt, and pepper.

3. Spread the dough onto a pizza sheet, bake, and check for golden crust. Rebake once toppings are added.

Curry soup made with chickpeas and vegetables
 Ingredients:
- 2 cans of rinsed and drained chickpeas
- A can of coconut milk
- A variety of chopped veggies, such as carrots, celery, and bell peppers
 - 2-tablespoon curry powder
 - Salt and pepper to taste

Make:
1. Saute vegetables in a big pot until they are soft.
2. Add salt, pepper, coconut milk, curry powder, and chickpeas. Simmer until thoroughly heated.

Soup with butternut squash and coconut:
Ingredients::
- 1 diced and peeled butternut squash
- 1 can coconut milk
- 1 chopped onion
- 2 minced garlic cloves
- 1 teaspoon curry powder
- Salt and pepper to taste

Make:
1. Soften the onion and garlic in a skillet.
2. Add enough water to cover the butternut squash, curry powder, and it. Cook the squash until it's soft.

3. Blend until smooth, adding coconut milk. Add salt and pepper to taste.

Avocado and Black Bean Salad:
Ingredients:
- 2 diced avocados
- 1 can washed and drained black beans
- 1 chopped red onion
- 1 cup halved cherry tomatoes
- Lime juice for the dressing and cilantro for garnish
- Salt and pepper to taste
Make:
1. Combine cherry tomatoes, red onion, black beans, and sliced avocado.

2. Add lime juice, salt, and pepper, and add cilantro as a garnish.

Rice and black beans with mango salsa:
Ingredients:
- 1 cup cooked rice
- 1 can washed and drained black beans
- 2 diced ripe mangos
- 1 diced red bell pepper
- 1/4 cup finely chopped red onion
- Fresh lime juice
- Garnishment of fresh cilantro

- Setting up:

1. Combine the cooked rice with the black beans, diced mangos, red onion, and red bell pepper.

2. Sprinkle cilantro on top and drizzle with fresh lime juice.

Risotto with spinach and mushrooms:
Ingredients:
- 1 1/2 cups Arborio rice
- 2 cups sliced mushrooms
- 4 cups of vegetable broth
- 2 cups of spinach
- 1 chopped onion
- 2 minced garlic cloves
- A optional 1/2 cup of white wine
- Oil of olives
- Pepper and salt to your liking

Preparation:

1. In olive oil, sauté onion and garlic until transparent.

2. Add the mushrooms and sauté them until the moisture is released.

3. Add the Arborio rice and stir. Cook for a couple of minutes.

4. Stirring until absorbed, gradually add the vegetable broth and white wine (if using).

5. When the spinach is wilted, add it along with salt and pepper.

Cucumber and Chickpea Salad
 Ingredients:
- 2 diced cucumbers
- 1 can of washed and drained chickpeas
- 1/4 cup coarsely chopped red onion
- 1/4 cup chopped fresh dill
 -2 tablespoons lemon juice
 - Oil of olives
- Salt and pepper to taste
Make:
1. Combine red onion, chopped cucumber, chickpeas, and fresh dill.

2. Add salt and pepper and drizzle with olive oil and lemon juice.

Portobello mushroom stuffing
 Ingredients include:
- Four sizable Portobello mushrooms.
- 1 cup cooked quinoa
- 1 cup chopped spinach
- Chopped half a cup of sun-dried tomatoes
- Optional 1/4 cup vegan cheese
- Oil of olives
- Salt and pepper to taste
Make:
1. Cut off the stems from the Portobello mushrooms and oil them.

2. Combine cooked quinoa, spinach that has been chopped, sun-dried tomatoes, and vegan cheese (if using) in a bowl.

3. Place the quinoa mixture inside each mushroom and bake the mushrooms until they are soft.

Broccoli with Stir-Fried Tofu:

Ingredients:
- 1 block diced firm tofu
- 2-cups of broccoli florets
- 2 tablespoons of gluten-free soy sauce
- 1-tablespoon rice vinegar
- 1-tablespoon maple syrup
- 1 teaspoon minced ginger
- 2 minced garlic cloves
- Sesame seeds for decoration
- Optional: Rice or rice noodles

- Setting up:

1. Combine soy sauce, maple syrup, rice vinegar, ginger, and garlic in a basin.

2. Stir-fry tofu in a hot skillet until it turns golden.

3. Combine the sauce mixture and broccoli. Cook broccoli until fork-tender.

4. Top with sesame seeds and serve with rice or rice noodles.

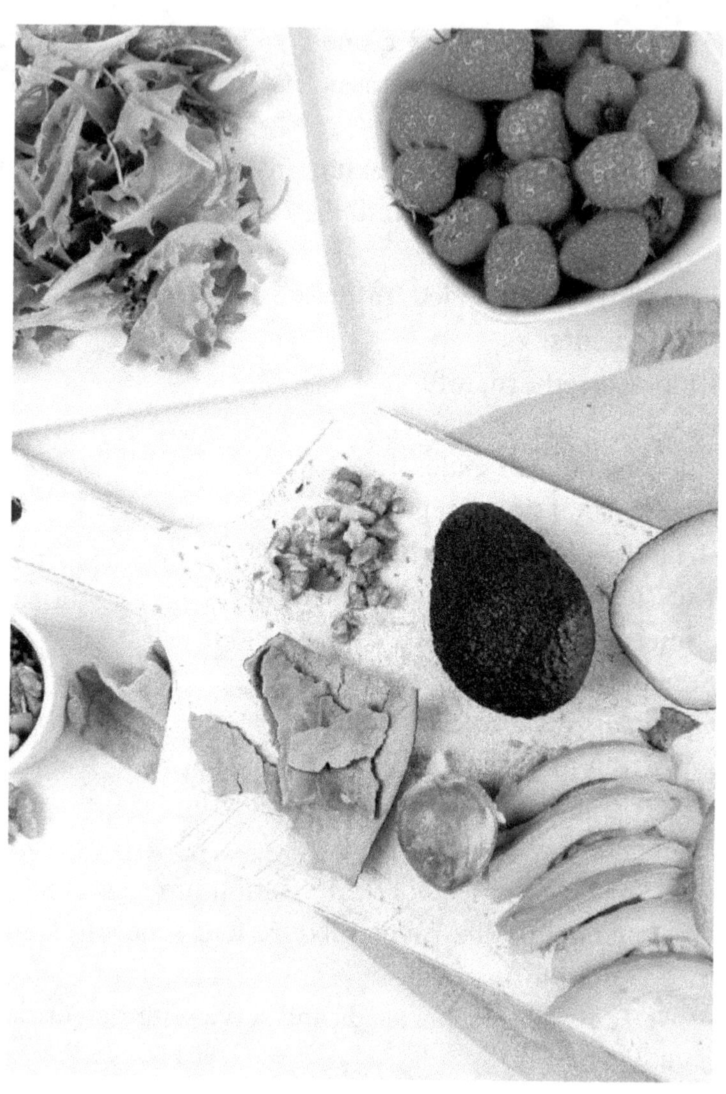

CHAPTER:10

Beverages

Classic Green Smoothie:
  - **Ingredients:**
    - 1 cup spinach leaves
    - 1/2 cup frozen banana
    - 1/2 cup almond milk
    - 1/2 cup water
    - 1 tablespoon honey (optional)
  Preparation:
Mix and blend all ingredients until smooth.

Blueberry Oatmeal Smoothie:
  - **Ingredients:**
    - 1 cup blueberries (fresh or frozen)
    - 1/2 cup rolled oats
    - 1 cup almond milk
    - 1 tablespoon maple syrup
  Preparation:
Blend until creamy.

Vegan Chocolate Shake:
  - **Ingredients:**
    - 1 cup almond milk
    - 2 tablespoons cocoa powder

- 2 tablespoons maple syrup
- 1/2 teaspoon vanilla extract

Preparation:

Blend all the ingredients until smooth.

Tropical Mango-Pineapple Smoothie:

- **Ingredients:**
  - 1 cup mango chunks
  - 1/2 cup pineapple chunks
  - 1/2 cup coconut milk
  - 1/2 cup orange juice

Preparation:

Blend until well combined.

Chai Latte:

- **Ingredients:**
  - 1 cup chai tea (brewed and cooled)
  - 1/2 cup almond milk
  - 1 tablespoon agave syrup
  - 1/4 teaspoon cinnamon

Preparation:

Mix all ingredients and warm them before serving.

Golden Milk Turmeric Latte:

- **Ingredients:**
  - 1 cup almond milk
  - 1 teaspoon turmeric powder
  - 1/2 teaspoon ginger powder

- 1 tablespoon maple syrup
Preparation:
Heat and whisk ingredients together.

Strawberry Banana Protein Smoothie:
- Ingredients:
  - 1 cup strawberries
  - 1 banana
  - 1/2 cup silken tofu
  - 1/2 cup almond milk
  - 1 tablespoon honey (optional)
Preparation:
Blend until creamy.

Cucumber Mint Cooler:
- Ingredients:
  - 1 cucumber (peeled and chopped)
  - 1/4 cup fresh mint leaves
  - 1/2 lemon (juiced)
  - 2 cups water
Preparation:
Blend and strain, then chill before serving.

Raspberry Lemonade:
- Ingredients:
  - 1 cup fresh raspberries
  - 1/2 cup lemon juice
  - 1/4 cup maple syrup

- 2 cups water

Preparation:

Blend and strain, serve over ice.

Coconut Water Mojito:

- **Ingredients:**
  - 1 cup coconut water
  - 1/2 lime (juiced)
  - 2 tablespoons fresh mint leaves
  - 1 tablespoon agave syrup

Preparation:

Muddle mint, add other ingredients, and stir.

Avocado and Kale Smoothie:

- **Ingredients:**
  - 1/2 avocado
  - 1 cup kale leaves
  - 1 banana
  - 1 cup almond milk
  - 1 tablespoon honey (optional)

Preparation:

Blend until creamy.

Pomegranate Blueberry Iced Tea:

- **Ingredients:**
  - 1 pomegranate tea bag
  - 1/2 cup blueberries
  - 1 tablespoon agave syrup

- Ice cubes

Preparation:

Brew tea, cool, and blend with blueberries and sweetener. Serve over ice.

Peach Almond Smoothie:
- **Ingredients:**
  - 2 ripe peaches (pitted)
  - 1/2 cup almond milk
  - 1/2 cup Greek yogurt (or dairy-free yogurt)
  - 1 tablespoon honey (optional)

  Preparation:

Blend until smooth.

Watermelon Cucumber Cooler:
- **Ingredients:**
  - 2 cups watermelon chunks
  - 1/2 cucumber (peeled and chopped)
  - 1/2 lime (juiced)
  - 1 tablespoon agave syrup

  Preparation:

Blend until well mixed.

Minty Iced Coffee
- **Ingredients:**
  - 1 cup brewed coffee (chilled)
  - 1/4 cup almond milk
  - 1/4 teaspoon peppermint extract

- 1 tablespoon agave syrup
Preparation:
Stir or shake all ingredients with ice.

Enjoy these refreshing plant-based beverage recipes!

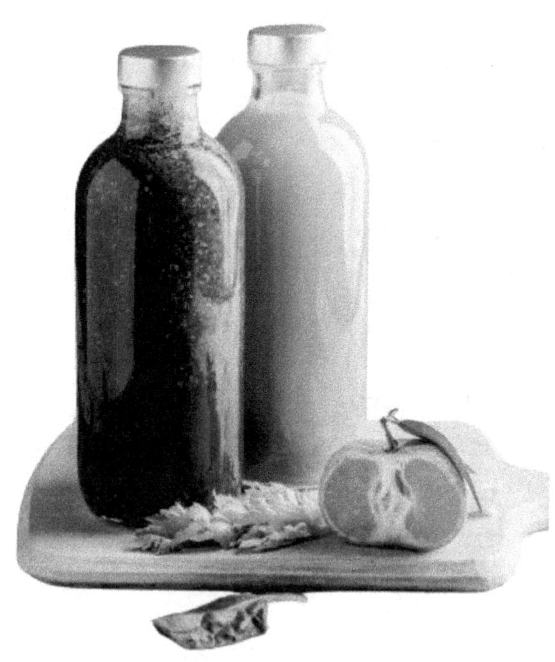

CHAPTER: 11

Desserts And Treats

Vegan Chocolate Avocado Mousse
  - **Ingredients:**
    - 2 ripe avocados
    - 1/4 cup cocoa powder
    - 1/4 cup maple syrup
    - 1 tsp vanilla extract
  Preparation:
   1. Blend all ingredients until smooth.
   2. Chill in the refrigerator for at least 30 minutes before serving.

Banana Ice Cream
  - **Ingredients:**
    - 4 ripe bananas, frozen
    - 1 tsp vanilla extract
  Preparation:
   1. Blend frozen bananas and vanilla extract until creamy.
   2. Serve immediately as soft-serve or freeze for a firmer texture.

Coconut Bliss Balls

- **Ingredients:**
  - 1 cup shredded coconut
  - 1/2 cup almond butter
  - 1/4 cup maple syrup
  - 1/4 cup chopped dark chocolate

Preparation:

1. Mix all ingredients together in a bowl.
2. Form into balls and chill until solid.

Chia Pudding

- **Ingredients:**
  - 1/4 cup chia seeds
  - 1 cup almond milk
  - 1 tbsp maple syrup
  - 1/2 tsp vanilla extract

Preparation:

1. Mix all ingredients, whisk well.
2. Refrigerate for at least 2 hours or overnight.

Vegan Berry Parfait

- **Ingredients:**
  - 1 cup mixed berries
  - 1 cup dairy-free yogurt
  - 1/4 cup granola

Preparation:

1. Layer yogurt, berries, and granola in a glass.

Avocado Lime Cheesecake

- **Ingredients:**
  - 2 ripe avocados
  - 1/4 cup lime juice
  - 1/4 cup maple syrup
  - 1 tsp vanilla extract

Preparation:

1. Blend avocados, lime juice, maple syrup, and vanilla until smooth.

2. Pour into a crust or glass dishes and refrigerate until set.

Vegan Chocolate Chip Cookies

- **Ingredients:**
  - 2 cups almond flour
  - 1/2 cup coconut oil
  - 1/2 cup maple syrup
  - 1/2 cup dairy-free chocolate chips

Preparation:

1. Mix almond flour, coconut oil, maple syrup, and chocolate chips.

2. Form into cookies and bake at 350°F (175°C) for 12-15 minutes.

Peanut Butter Energy Bites

- **Ingredients:**
  - 1 cup oats
  - 1/2 cup peanut butter

- 1/4 cup maple syrup
- 1/4 cup chopped dates
- **Preparation:**
  1. Mix all ingredients.
  2. Form into bite-sized balls, then chill.

Vegan Rice Pudding

- **Ingredients:**
  - 1 cup cooked rice
  - 2 cups coconut milk
  - 1/4 cup maple syrup
  - 1 tsp vanilla extract
- **Preparation:**
  1. Combine all ingredients in a saucepan and simmer until thickened.

Mango Sorbet

- **Ingredients:**
  - 2 ripe mangoes, peeled and chopped
  - 2 tbsp lime juice
  - 1/4 cup agave nectar
- **Preparation:**
  1. Blend mangoes, lime juice, and agave nectar.
  2. Freeze until firm.

Chocolate Avocado Truffles

- **Ingredients:**
  - 2 ripe avocados

- 1/2 cup cocoa powder

- 1/4 cup maple syrup

- Preparation:

1. Blend avocados, cocoa powder, and maple syrup until smooth.

2. Roll into truffles and chill.

Vegan Apple Crisp

- Ingredients:

- 4 apples, peeled and sliced

- 1 cup oats

- 1/2 cup almond flour

- 1/4 cup maple syrup

- Preparation:

1. Mix apples with a bit of maple syrup and place in a baking dish.

2. Combine oats, almond flour, and maple syrup, then sprinkle over the apples.

3. Bake at 350°F (175°C) for 30 minutes.

Chickpea Chocolate Chip Blondies

- Ingredients:

- 1 can chickpeas, drained and rinsed

- 1/2 cup almond butter

- 1/4 cup maple syrup

- 1 tsp vanilla extract

- 1/2 cup dairy-free chocolate chips

- Preparation:

1. Blend chickpeas, almond butter, maple syrup, and vanilla until smooth.

2. Stir in chocolate chips, then bake in an 8x8-inch pan at 350°F (175°C) for 20-25 minutes.

Pumpkin Pie Smoothie

- Ingredients:

- 1 cup pumpkin puree
- 1 cup almond milk
- 1 banana
- 1 tsp pumpkin spice
- 1 tbsp maple syrup

- Preparation:

1. Blend all ingredients until smooth.

Vegan Chocolate Pudding

- Ingredients:

- 1/2 cup silken tofu
- 1/4 cup cocoa powder
- 1/4 cup maple syrup
- 1 tsp vanilla extract

- Preparation:

1. Blend tofu, cocoa powder, maple syrup, and vanilla until creamy.

2. Before serving, chill in the fridge.

Blueberry Oat Bars

  - **Ingredients:**
    - 2 cups rolled oats
    - 1 cup blueberries
    - 1/4 cup maple syrup
    - 1/4 cup almond butter
  - **Preparation:**
    1. Mix oats, blueberries, maple syrup, and almond butter.
    2. Press into a baking dish and bake at 350°F (175°C) for 25-30 minutes.

Vegan Tiramisu

  - **Ingredients:**
    - 1 package vegan ladyfingers
    - 1 cup brewed coffee
    - 1 cup cashew cream (blended cashews and water)
    - 1/4 cup cocoa powder
  - **Preparation:**
    1. Dip ladyfingers in coffee and layer in a dish.
    2. Spread cashew cream over the ladyfingers.
    3. Dust with cocoa powder and chill.

Vegan Lemon Bars

  - **Ingredients:**
    - 1 cup almond flour
    - 1/4 cup lemon juice
    - 1/4 cup maple syrup

- Zest of one lemon
  - **Preparation:**
    1. Mix almond flour, lemon juice, maple syrup, and lemon zest.
    2. Press into a dish and bake at 350°F (175°C) for 20-25 minutes.

Chocolate-Dipped Strawberries
  - **Ingredients:**
    - Fresh strawberries
    - Vegan chocolate chips, melted
  - **Preparation:**
    1. Dip strawberries in melted chocolate.
    2. Place on a tray and refrigerate until the chocolate sets.

Pumpkin Spice Energy Balls
  - **Ingredients:**
    - 1 cup rolled oats
    - 1/2 cup pumpkin puree
    - 1/4 cup almond butter
    - 1/4 cup maple syrup
    - 1 tsp pumpkin spice
  - **Preparation:**
    1. Mix all ingredients.
    2. Roll into balls and refrigerate.

Enjoy making these delicious plant-based desserts and treats!

CONCLUSION

The plant-based diet cookbook is a potent tool for altering our health, the environment, and our culinary experiences. It is more than just a compilation of recipes. This cookbook's pages have opened our eyes to the wide variety of tastes, textures, and nutritional advantages that may be obtained from the abundant supply of plants that Mother Earth supplies.

This cookbook offers proof of the adaptability and innovation of plant-based cuisine. We now know that plant-based cuisine is capable of producing meals that are as scrumptious, savory, and varied as any other. This cookbook has something for everyone, regardless of whether you're a seasoned vegan or just starting out on your plant-based eating path. It's an important tool for people who want to increase their intake of nutrient-dense plants while decreasing their use of animal products.

This cookbook also highlights the crucial part that everyone of us must play in reducing the negative effects that our food choices have on the environment. We can lower greenhouse gas emissions, preserve water supplies, and safeguard biodiversity by switching to a plant-based diet. This cookbook's recipes are all little steps in the direction of a more sustainable future.

This cookbook is a celebration of the joy of cooking and eating, which is possibly its most significant aspect. It serves as a reminder that food serves as more than just a source of energy for us; it also fosters relationships, culture, and enjoyment. This cookbook invites us to gather around the table, share healthful meals with loved ones, and savor the beauty of plant-based food via the colorful and delectable dishes it provides.

The plant-based diet cookbook is a ray of hope and a manual for adopting a more kindhearted and environmentally conscious diet in a world where environmental and health issues are becoming increasingly pressing. It gives us the ability to make decisions that are beneficial for not only our own health but also the health of the planet and future generations. So let's grab our aprons, get to the kitchen, and start experimenting with more delicious plant-based recipes to discover the countless possibilities of this method of cooking.